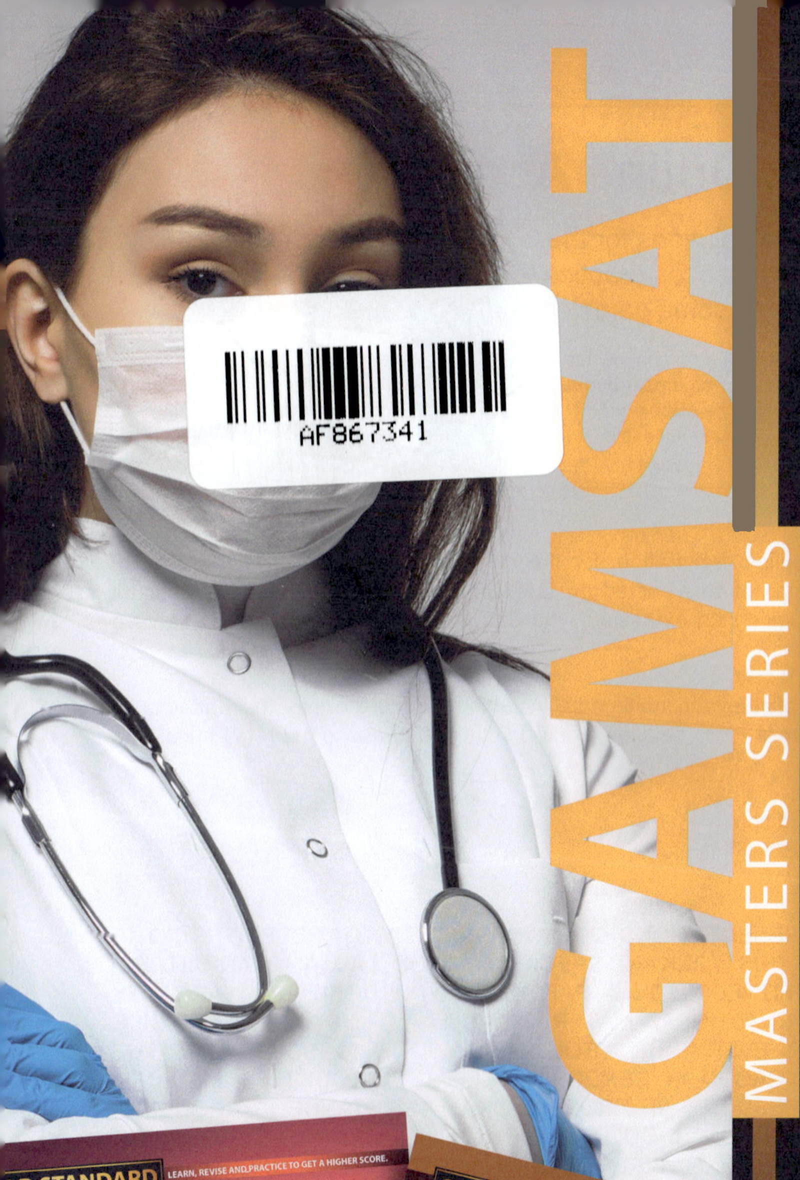

GOLD STANDARD

PERMISSION GRANTED

If you wish to share your study experience in social media (e.g. Instagram, TikTok, YouTube, etc.), Gold Standard GAMSAT gives you the permission to include any of our books (cover and/or interior pages, though never all pages from a chapter), and/or short segments of our videos, in your content. Share your study journey and inspire others!

01 **Editor and Author**
Brett Ferdinand BSc MD-CM

02 **Contributors**
Lisa Ferdinand BA MA
Sean Pierre BSc MD
Kristin Finkenzeller BSc MD
Ibrahima Diouf BSc MSc PhD
Charles Haccoun BSc MD-CM
Timothy Ruger BA MA
Jeanne Tan Te

03 **Illustrators**
Harvie W. Gallatiera BS CompE
Gilbert Rafanan BSc

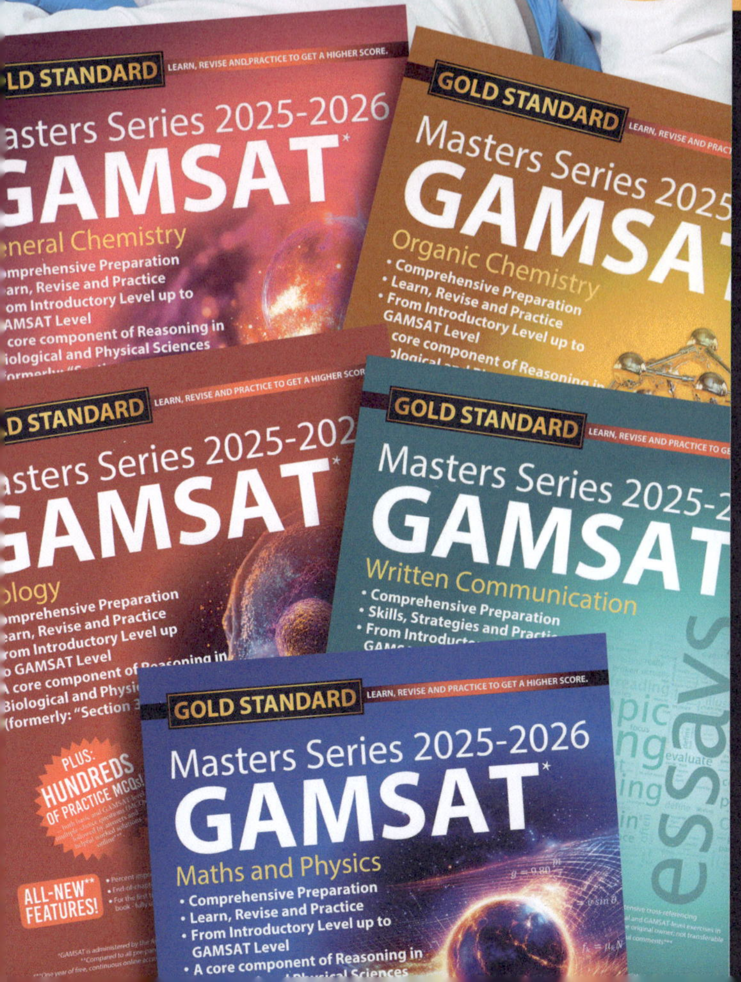

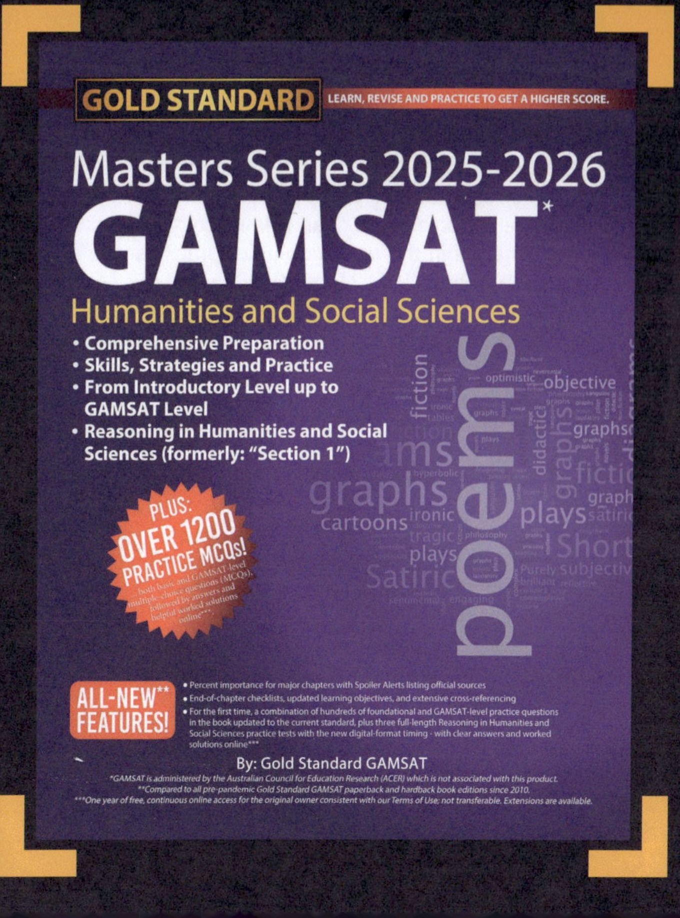

Register your book!

Free Online Access*

Answers and worked solutions for the 3 full-length Reasoning in Humanities and Social Sciences practice tests at the back of the book and some sample videos.

*One year of continuous access for the original owner of this textbook upon online registration at www.gamsat-prep.com/gamsat-humanities-and-social-sciences
If you purchased this textbook or the eBook directly from www.gamsat-prep.com, then your online access is automated.

Please note: Benefits last for one year from the date of online registration, for the original book owner only, and are not transferable; unauthorized access and use outside the Terms of Use posted on GAMSAT-prep.com may result in account deletion; if you are not the original owner, or if you are seeking an extension, you can purchase your virtual access card separately at GAMSAT-prep.com.

Online access: reduces digital piracy; allows the addition of relevant multimedia including videos; permits the updating of strategies and content to reflect the evolving GAMSAT; permits more detailed worked solutions; reduces the retail price; and ultimately, saves trees!

ISBN 978-1-927338-88-9

Address all inquiries, comments, or suggestions to the publisher. For Terms of Use go to: www.GAMSAT-prep.com

Gold Standard GAMSAT Product Contact Information

Distribution in Australia, NZ, Asia

Woodslane Pty Ltd 10 Apollo Street
Warriewood NSW 2102 Australia
ABN: 76 003 677 549
learn@gamsat-prep.com

Distribution in Europe

Central Books 99 Wallis
Road LONDON,
E9 5LN, United Kingdom
orders@centralbooks.com

Distribution in North America

RuveneCo Publishing
334 Cornelia Street #559
Plattsburgh, New York 12901, USA
buy@gamsatbooks.com

GAMSAT (Graduate Medical School Admissions Test)

Computer-based exam held at test centres internationally for graduate-entry medicine

Written Communication (Writing Tasks A & B)

- formerly "Section 2"

2 essays responding to 2 different themes using sound reasoning and competent English-writing skills (essays must be typed)

Writing Task A: sociocultural theme (e.g., free speech, justice, social media)
Writing Task B: personal-social themes (e.g., humour, love, happiness)

Reasoning in Humanities and Social Sciences

- formerly "Section 1"

multiple-choice section with stimulus materials requiring comprehension and analysis of non-science content

poetry • proverbs • cartoons • novels or play excerpts • travel and/or medical journal entries • social science graphs

Reasoning in Biological and Physical Sciences

- formerly "Section 3"

multiple-choice section with questions mostly based on science passages that require problem-solving and graph analysis

first-year undergraduate level Biology (40%), General Chemistry (20%) & Organic Chemistry (20%) • A-level/Leaving Certificate/ Year 12 level Physics (20%)

Top GAMSAT Score: 100
Average GAMSAT Score: 57

Summary of the new Digital-format GAMSAT Exam Day

	KEY POINTS	EVENT	DURATION
Written Communication	Produce ideas in writing with clarity and soundness; essays are typed with no copy/paste function	2 essays typed on a computer (for all sections including the essays: no longer is there a formal, dedicated reading time)	65 minutes
Arrival and Sitting of Exam	Bring only the acceptable ID documents and permitted items to the test centre as specified in ACER's GAMSAT Information Booklet	Security, identification, health protocols	15-45 minutes
Reasoning in Humanities and Social Sciences	Key skills are reading speed and comprehension of information within socio-cultural contexts	62 MCQs* (the test centre will provide you with 2 sheets of A4 scratch paper; *option*: whiteboard)	100 minutes
Break	Consider packing your own lunch to avoid queues with nervous chatter	–	20 minutes
Reasoning in Biological and Physical Sciences	Analyse and solve problems: 40% Biology, 40% Chemistry (equally split between General and Organic); 20% Physics	75 MCQs* (the test centre will provide you with 2 new sheets of A4 scratch paper; *option*: whiteboard)	150 minutes
Total Test Time	Success requires stamina; stamina improves with practice.	–	5 hours, 15 minutes

*MCQs: multiple-choice questions, 4 options per question with only 1 best answer. Note that the 'old' GAMSAT had a dedicated 'reading time' of 10 minutes for each of Section 1 and 3, and 5 minutes for Section 2. During that reading time, students were not permitted to write or mark their exam paper in any way. The new digital GAMSAT has added time for each of the 3 exam sections as a legacy to 'reading time'; however, in practice, you can use your exam time in any way that you see fit.

**It might be a good idea to allocate a whole day to sit the GAMSAT test to allow for any contingencies and/or technical issues that you might encounter. Safety measures and health protocols should be carefully anticipated when making travel arrangements and accommodations to and from the testing centre.

Common formula for acceptance:

GPA + GAMSAT score + Interview = Medical School Admissions

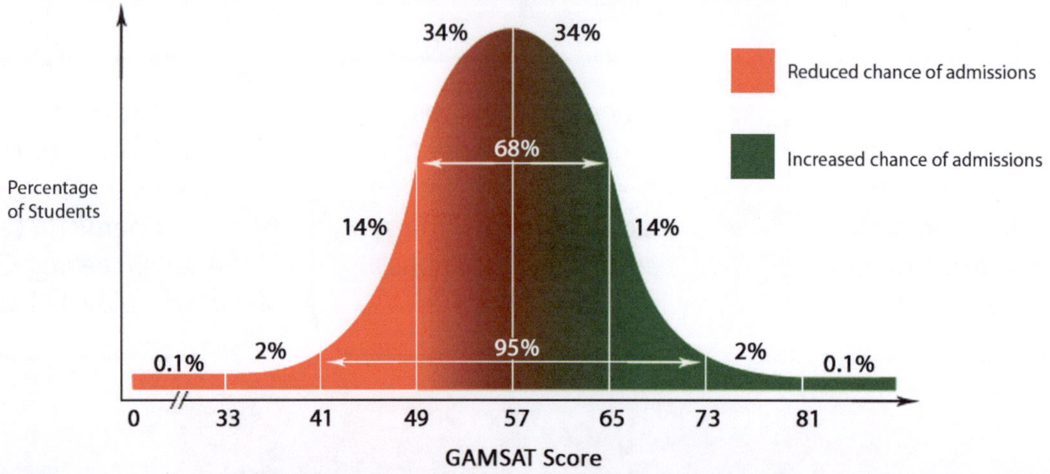

Typical Overall GAMSAT Score Distribution (Approx)

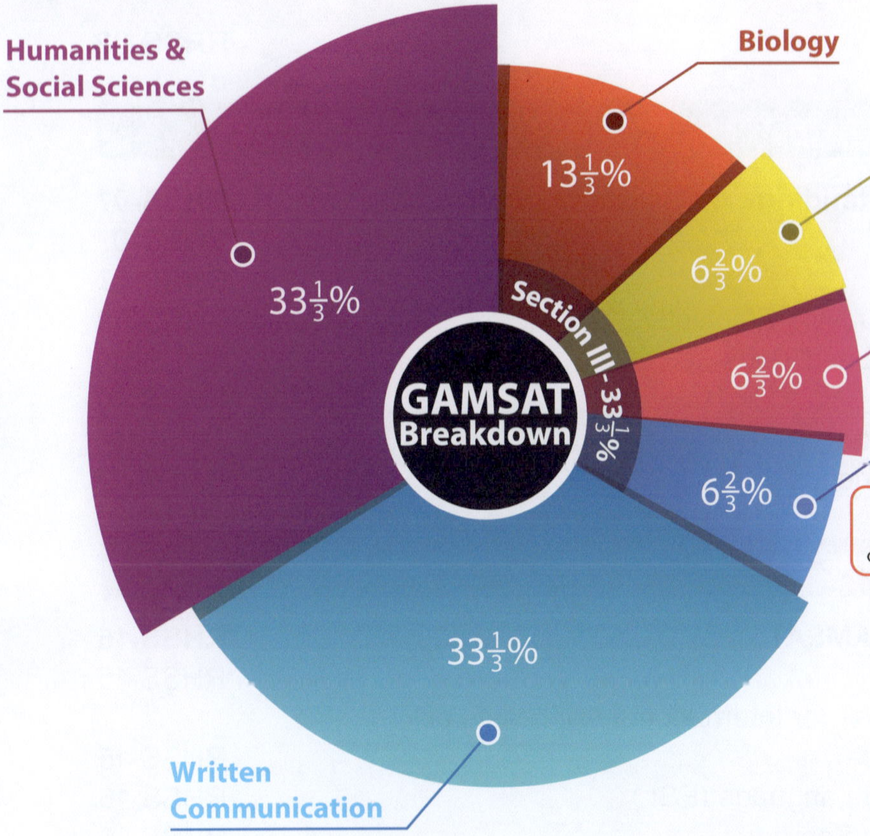

Please note: Some medical schools weigh all 3 sections equally, as illustrated in the pie chart to the left, while others weigh Section III (the sciences) twice as seen below.

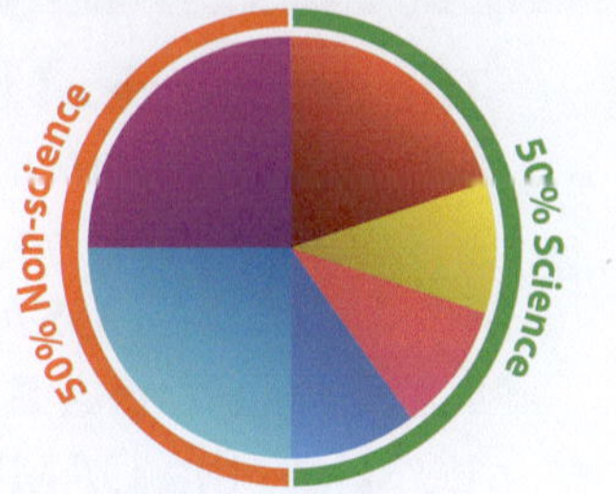

GAMSAT is challenging, get organised.

gamsat-prep.com/free-GAMSAT-study-schedule

1. How to study

- Learn, revise and practice using the GAMSAT Masters Series book(s) and/or videos.
- Complete all exercises and multiple-choice practice questions in this book.
- Consolidate: create and study from your personal summaries (= Gold Notes) daily. Create study cards or audio files from your Gold Notes to increase your study efficiency.

2. Once you have completed your studies

- Sit a full-length GAMSAT practice test.
- Analyse mistakes and all worked solutions.
- Consolidate; Revise all your Gold Notes and create more.

3. Sit multiple mock exams

- ACER GAMSAT practice exams with free Gold Standard worked solutions on YouTube
- Free full-length Gold Standard (GS) mock exam GS-Free with helpful, detailed worked solutions
- HEAPS: 15 full-length exams, 5 in the book and 10 online with the new, digital GAMSAT format

4. How much time do you need to study?

- On average, 3-6 hours per day for 3-6 months; depending on life experiences, 2 weeks may be enough and 8 months could be insufficient.
- Try to study full on for 1-2 weeks and then adjust your expectations for your personal, ideal study time.

5. Recommended GAMSAT Communities

- All countries (mainly Australia): pagingdr.net
- Mainly the UK: thestudentroom.co.uk (Medicine Community Discussion)
- Mainly Ireland: boards.ie (GAMSAT and GEM forum)

Is there something in the Masters Series that you did not understand? Don't get frustrated, get online:

gamsat-prep.com/forum

Note that: H = High-level Importance; M = Medium-level Importance; L = Low-level Importance.

Note that: H = High-level Importance; M = Medium-level Importance; L = Low-level Importance.

INTRODUCTION

Let's discuss medical school admissions!

Patients and medical professionals often point to three key characteristics of a successful doctor: knowledge, reasoning and interpersonal skills. Clearly, in order to successfully treat illness, knowledge of the condition and treatment options is important. However, reasoning is required to distil all that is possible down to the most likely diagnosis and create an appropriate plan. Despite the preceding, the patient may not want to comply with treatment if interpersonal skills are lacking.

The medical school admissions process has been designed - in part - to address societal concerns. To determine if you are capable of acquiring knowledge at the agreed standard, your GPA is examined. This reflects the sad reality that the majority of undergraduate studies focus more on memory and less so on higher-order thinking skills. But here comes the GAMSAT! The first word in the description of both GAMSAT multiple-choice sections is "Reasoning." Once you start practicing, you will quickly see how memory is downplayed and reasoning is elevated.

The medical school interview - in particular, the MMI (multiple mini-interview) - was born to address the issue of interpersonal skills. Of course, the skills required for the 3 main criteria of medical school admissions overlap to some degree.

In summary, your GPA and GAMSAT score can write the ticket for a medical school interview where success opens the door for admissions. Our aim is to be of help every step of the way. We have created a permanently-free section in your gamsat-prep.com account with hours of helpful medical school interview videos exploring important strategies. The Masters Series books now have the most accurate and up-to-date GAMSAT practice questions ever assembled.

In the first section of this book, we begin with a concise examination as to how you can improve your grades at school; even if you have finished your formal studies, you will find some of the advice helpful to improve your study efficiency during your GAMSAT preparation.

The next section of the book, 'Understanding the GAMSAT', takes a closer look at the structure of the exam, strategies for all sections, and how to continue to plan your preparation moving forward.

And finally, the bulk of this book exists for the real reason that you are here: To learn the vocabulary, ideas, and strategies to optimise your GAMSAT score. As part of your coaching, we have prepared over 1200 foundational and GAMSAT-standard practice questions in Reasoning in Humanities and Social Sciences (RHSS, formerly known as "Section 1"). We will explore all of the above, together, comprehensively, and practice, extensively. We start with simple ideas and then we work up to GAMSAT-level reasoning. Whatever your skill level, you will be able to acclimatise to the challenge while developing and/or expanding your English skills.

For the entirety of this book, please consider the mantra: *practice, practice, practice.*

Good luck with your studies!

– BF, MD

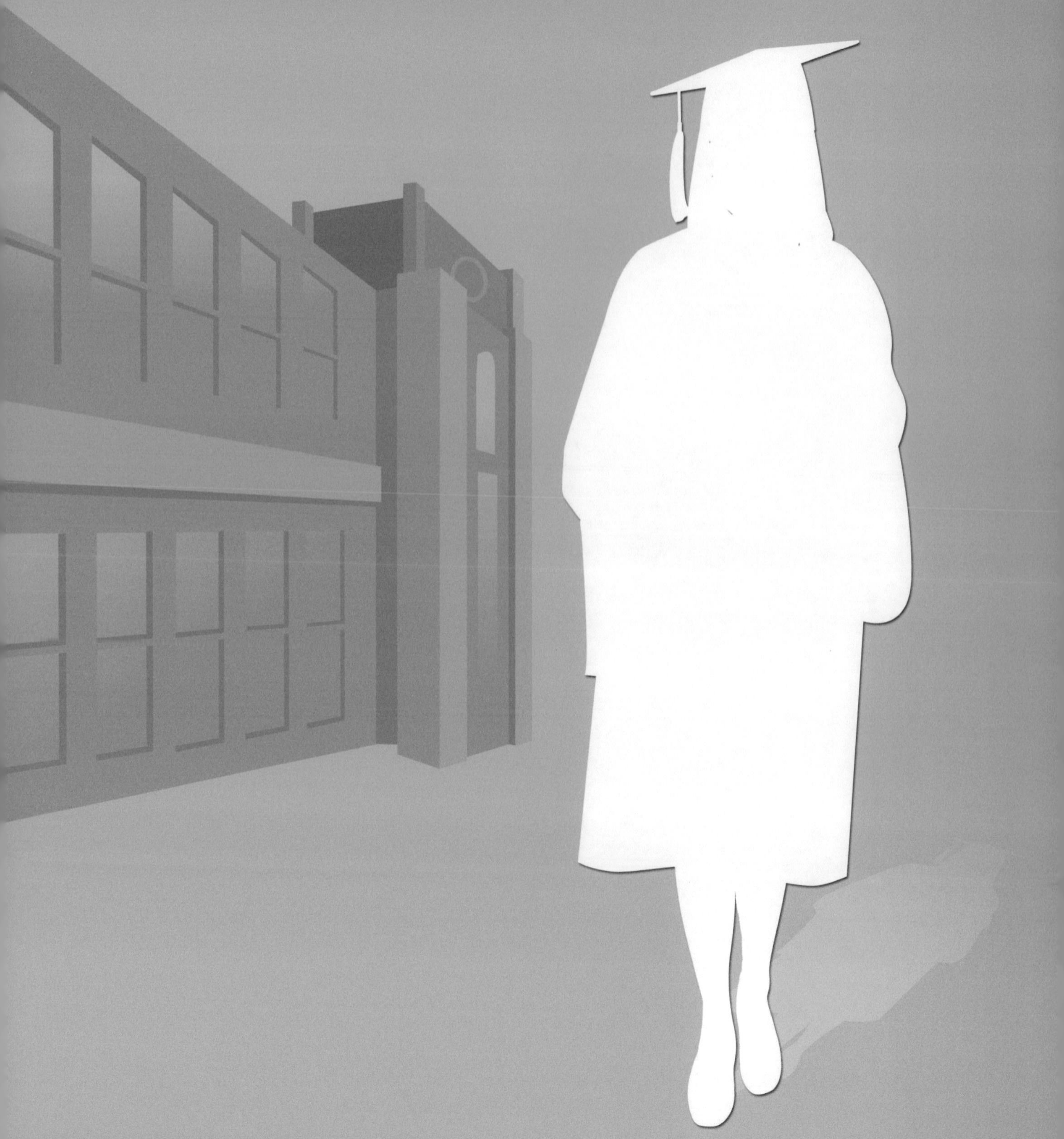

GAMSAT-Prep.com

MEDICAL SCHOOL ADMISSIONS

PART I

IMPROVING ACADEMIC STANDING

1.1 Lectures

Before you set foot in a classroom you should consider the value of being there. Even if you were taking a course like 'Basket-weaving 101', one way to help you do well in the course is to consider the value of the course to **you**. The course should have an *intrinsic* value (i.e. 'I enjoy weaving baskets'). The course will also have an *extrinsic* value (i.e. 'If I do not get good grades, I will not be accepted...'). Motivation, a positive attitude, and an interest in learning give you an edge before the class even begins.

Unless there is a student 'note-taking club' for your courses, your attendance record and the quality of your notes should both be as excellent as possible. Be sure to choose seating in the classroom which ensures that you will be able to hear the professor adequately and see whatever she may write. Whenever possible, do not sit close to friends!

Instead of chattering before the lecture begins, spend the idle moments quickly studying from your notes from the previous lecture in that subject so you would have an idea of what to expect. Try to take good notes and pay close attention. The preceding may sound like a difficult combination (esp. with professors who speak and write quickly); however, with practice you can learn to do it well.

And finally, do not let the quality of teaching affect your interest in the subject nor your grades! Do not waste your time during or before lectures complaining about how the professor speaks too quickly, does not explain concepts adequately, etc... When the time comes, you can mention such issues on the appropriate evaluation forms! In the meantime, consider this: despite the good or poor quality of teaching, there is always a certain number of students who **still** perform well. You must strive to count yourself among those students.

1.2 Taking Notes

Unless your professor says otherwise, if you take excellent notes and master those notes, you will *ace* his course. Your notes should always be up-to-date, complete, and separate from other subjects.

To be safe, you should try to write everything! You can fill in any gaps by comparing your notes with those of your friends. If you do not type then create your own shorthand symbols or use standard ones. The following represents some useful symbols:

|·|	*between*
=	*the same as*
≠	*not the same as*
∴	*therefore*
Δ	*difference, change in*
cf.	*compare*
c̄ or w	*with*
c̄out or w/o	*without*
esp.	*especially*
∵	*because*
i.e.	*that is*
e.g.	*for example*

Many students retype or rewrite their notes at home. Should you decide to rewrite your notes, your time will be used efficiently if you are paying close attention to the information you are rewriting. In fact, a more useful technique is the following: during class, write your notes only on the right side of your binder. Later, rewrite the information from class in a complete but condensed form on the left side of the binder (*this condensed form should include mnemonics which we will discuss later*). If you retype, again, your focus should be to condense your notes (this requires that you continually decide what you already know).

The advice for taking notes (condensed with symbols) applies to your study of the Masters Series books as it does to the note-taking that you may do during the new, digital GAMSAT. The test centre will provide you with two A4 sheets to be used as scratch paper.

1.3 The Principles of Studying Efficiently

If you study efficiently, you will have enough time to work, and/or study for the GAMSAT, and/or pursue university studies. The bottom line is that your time must be used efficiently and effectively. Note that the following advice applies to full-time students as well as those of you with full-time employment seeking ways to study more efficiently for the GAMSAT.

In school: During the average school day, time can be found during breaks, between classes, and after school to quickly revise your notes in a library or any other quiet place you can find on campus. Simply by using the available time in your school day, you can keep up-to-date with recent information.

At work: Most jobs have some downtime during the day. Coffee breaks, lunch, miscellaneous waiting time, are all opportunities for study. Any time spent in a vehicle or public transportation may represent hours of extra study time per week with study aids such as MP3s (section 1.5).

When you sign in to your gamsat-prep.com account, you will notice a button for "GAMSAT Study Schedule" which presents an intense programme with day-by-day suggested goals. You can follow that schedule, or preferably, modify it according to your own needs. As a rule, a certain amount of time every evening should be set aside for more in depth studying. Weekends can be set aside for special projects and revising notes from the beginning.

On the surface, the idea of regularly revising notes from the beginning may sound like an insurmountable task which would take forever! The reality is just the opposite. After all, if you continually study the information, by the time the real GAMSAT or mid-terms approach, you would have seen your first set of notes so many times that it would take only moments to revise it again. On the other hand, had you not been revising regularly, it would be like reading those notes for the first time!

You should study wherever you are <u>comfortable</u> and <u>effective</u> studying (i.e. library, at home, etc.). Should you prefer studying at home, be sure to create an environment which is conducive to studying.

Studying should be an active process to <u>memorise</u> and <u>understand</u> a given set of material. Memorisation and comprehension are best achieved by the **elaboration** of course material, **attention, repetition,** and practising **retrieval** of the information. All these principles are borne out in the following techniques.

1.4 Studying from Notes and Texts

Successful studying from either class notes, university textbooks, or GAMSAT Masters Series textbooks, can be accomplished in three simple steps:

- **Preview the material**: read all the relevant headings, titles, and subtitles to give you a general idea of what you are about to learn. You should never embark on a trip without knowing where you are going! Note that all GAMSAT Masters Series books are organised by section and subsection. Before reading the chapter from the beginning, survey the entire chapter by looking at all of the headings and glimpse graphs, tables or diagrams.

- **Read while questioning**: **<u>passive studying</u>** is when you sit in front of a book and just read. This can lead to boredom, lack of concentration, or even worse - difficulty remembering what you just read! **<u>Active studying</u>** involves reading while actively questioning yourself. For example: how does this fit in with the 'big picture'? How does this relate to what I learned last week? What cues about these words or lists will make it easy for me to memorise them? What type of question would ACER or my professor ask me? If I was asked a question on this material, how would I answer? Etc...

- **Recite and consider**: put the notes or text away while you attempt to **recall** the main facts. Once you are able to recite the important information, **consider** how it relates to the entire subject.

N.B. if you ever sit down to study and you are not quite sure with which subject to begin, always start with either the most difficult subject or the subject you like least (usually they are one and the same!).

1.5 Study Aids

The most effective study aids include practice exams, mnemonics, audio MP3s and study cards.

Practice exams (*exams from previous semesters*) are often available online or directly from the professor. They can be used like maps which guide you through your semester. They give you a good indication as to what information you should emphasise when you study; what question types and exam format you can expect; and what your level of progress is.

One practice exam should be set aside to sit one week before 'the real thing.' You should time yourself and sit the exam in an environment free from distractions. This provides an ideal way to uncover unexpected weak points. {We will have a discussion about GAMSAT practice tests in the next section of this book: 2.1, The Recipe for GAMSAT Success.}

Mnemonics are an effective way of memorising lists of information. Usually a word, phrase, or sentence is constructed to symbolise a greater amount of information (i.e. LEO is A GERC = Lose Electrons is Oxidation is Anode, Gain Electrons is Reduction at Cathode). An effective study aid to active studying is the creation of your own mnemonics.

Audio MP3s (e.g., audio files or 'voice memos') can be used as effective tools to repeat information and to use your time efficiently. Information from the left side of your notes (*see 1.2 Taking Notes*) including mnemonics, can be dictated and recorded. Often, an entire semester of work can be summarised into one 90-minute recording.

Now you can listen to the recording on your smartphone while waiting in line at the bank, or in a bus or with a car stereo on the way to school, work, etc. You can also listen to recorded information when you go to sleep and listen to another one first thing in the morning. You are probably familiar with the situation of having heard a song early in the morning and then having difficulty, for the rest of the day, getting it out of your mind! Well, imagine if the first thing you heard in the morning was: "Organic Chemistry nomenclature: 3 carbons uses the prefix prop- such as the ketone propanone AKA acetone..."! Thus MP3s become an effective study aid since they are an extra source of repetition.

Some students like to use **study cards** (tangible flashcards and/or smartphone apps) on which they may write either a summary of information they must memorise or relevant questions to consider. Then the cards are used throughout the day to quickly flash information to promote thought on course material.

1.5.1 Falling Behind

Imagine yourself as a marathon runner who has run 25.5 km of a 26 km race. The finishing line is now in view. However, you have fallen behind some of the other runners. The most difficult aspect of the race is still ahead.

In such a scenario some interesting questions can be asked: Is now the time to drop out of the race because 0.5 km suddenly seems like a long distance? Is now the time to reevaluate whether or not you should have competed? Or is now the time to remain faithful to your goals and give 100%?

Imagine one morning in mid-semester you wake up realising you have fallen behind in your studies. What do you do? Where do you start? Is it too late?

Like a doctor being presented with an urgent matter, you should see the situation as one of life's challenges. Now is the worst time for doubts, rather, it is the time for action. A clear line of action should be formulated such that it could be followed.

For example, one might begin by gathering all pertinent study materials like a complete set of study notes, relevant text(s), sample exams, etc. As a rule, to get back into the thick of things, notes and sample exams take precedence. Studying at this point should take a three-pronged approach: i) a regular, consistent study of the information from your notes from the beginning of the section for which you are responsible (i.e. *starting with the first class*); ii) a regular, consistent study of course material as you are learning it from the lectures (*this is the most efficient way to study*); iii) regular testing using questions given in class or those contained in sample exams. Using such questions will clarify the extent of your progress.

It is also of value, as time allows, to engage in extracurricular activities which you find helpful in reducing stress (i.e. sports, piano, creative writing, etc.).

1.5.2 Family and Friends

Your family and friends can be tremendous study aids or they can, let's say, be the source of significant challenges. Of course, it may be difficult for those who feel close to you to lose access to you because of your studies.

Let your family and friends know, early and often, about your objective (e.g. medicine, a successful GAMSAT score) and explain what that entails. They will be more likely to encourage you and less likely to distract you if they understand that you will be less available for a limited time because of an admirable goal.

$$\mathcal{A} + \mathcal{B} = ?$$

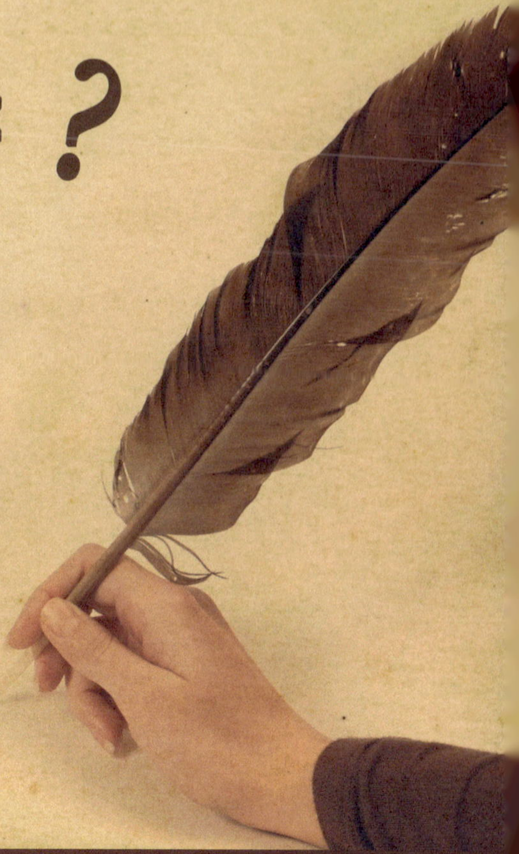

GAMSAT-Prep.com

UNDERSTANDING THE GAMSAT

PART II

THE STRUCTURE OF THE GAMSAT

1.1 Introduction

The Graduate Medical School Admissions Test (GAMSAT) is a prerequisite for admission to participating graduate-entry professional programmes including medical and dental schools in Australia, Ireland and the UK. Each year thousands of applicants submit GAMSAT test results to medical, dental and graduate schools as well as other programmes (i.e. pharmacy, optometry, veterinary science, etc.). While the actual weight given to GAMSAT scores in the admissions process varies from school to school, often they are regarded in a similar manner to your university GPA (i.e. your academic standing).

The GAMSAT is available to any student who has already completed a bachelor's degree, or who will be enrolled in their penultimate (second to last) or final year of study for a bachelor's degree, at the time of sitting the test. The test is administered twice a year, in March and September, at test centres in Australia, the UK and Ireland. The March sitting and September sitting are no longer referred to as 'GAMSAT Australia/ Ireland' or 'GAMSAT UK,' respectively, since each sitting is now available in all three countries. Not all test centres are offered for each sitting. Additional test centres are available in Singapore, Washington D.C. (USA), and Wellington (NZ).

GAMSAT results are generally valid for 2 years. There is no restriction on the number of times you may sit the GAMSAT. Currently, results from sitting the GAMSAT in any one country can be used in applying to any other country that requires the GAMSAT.

To access the most up-to-date information, to register for the GAMSAT, and to purchase official GAMSAT practice materials, consider visiting the following website: gamsat.acer.org.

1.1.1 The *new* MCAT for International Applicants or for US/Canada

The new Medical College Admission Test (MCAT) is a prerequisite for admission to nearly all the medical schools in North America. Each year, over 50,000 applicants to American and English Canadian medical schools submit MCAT test results.

The MCAT is a computer-based test (CBT) administered on a Saturday or a weekday, more than 20 times per year. To register for the MCAT, you should consult your undergraduate adviser and register online: www.aamc.org.

The MCAT can be used by international students applying to medical schools that accept GAMSAT scores. Only international students have the option of sitting the MCAT instead of the GAMSAT. Consult individual programmes for confirmation.

1.2 English as a Second Language (ESL)

Many ESL students will need to pay extra attention to Written Communication (WC) and Reasoning in Humanities and Social Sciences (RHSS) of the GAMSAT. Specific advice for all students will be presented in the chapters that follow. This advice should be taken very seriously for ESL students.

Having said that, GAMSAT scores are subjected to a statistical analysis to check that each question is fair, valid and reliable. Test questions in development are scrutinised in order to minimise gender, ethnic or religious bias, in order to affirm that the test is culturally fair.

Candidates whose native language is not English are permitted to bring a printed bilingual dictionary on test day for use in WC and RHSS only. The pages must be unmarked and all paper notes removed. Any candidate using this option must submit the dictionary to the Supervisor for inspection before the test begins.

Depending on your English skills, you may or may not benefit from an English reading or writing summer course. Of course, you would have the option of deciding whether or not you would want to take such a course for credit. Your online account at GAMSAT-prep.com comes with dozens of speed reading and comprehension exercises ranging from very basic up to GAMSAT-level practice.

1.3 How the GAMSAT is Scored

The GAMSAT is scored for each of the three sections individually. The sections consisting of multiple-choice questions are first scored right or wrong resulting in a raw score. Note that wrong answers are worth the same as unanswered questions so ALWAYS ANSWER ALL THE QUESTIONS even if you are not sure of certain answers. The raw score is then converted to a scaled score ranging from 0 (lowest) to 100 (highest). Essentially, the scores are scaled to ensure that the same proportion of individual marks within each section are given from year to year (using Item Response Theory). The scaled score is neither a percentage nor a percentile. It is not possible to accurately replicate this scoring system at home.

Written Communication (WC, 2 essays) is marked by three independent markers from each zone. A scale of 10 points is used. Should there be a difference of 5 or more in two scores then an additional marker will be used. Ultimately, the three closest scores are totaled for the Written Communication raw score which is then converted to a scaled score.

You will receive a score for each of the three sections, together with an Overall GAMSAT Score. The Overall Score is a weighted average of the three component scores.

The Overall GAMSAT Score is determined using the following formula:

Overall Score = (1 × WC + 1 × RHSS + 2 × Sciences) ÷ 4

Standards for interviews or admissions may vary for both Sectional Scores and the Overall GAMSAT Score. For example, one particular medical school may establish a cut-off (minimum) of 50 for any given section and 60 for the Overall GAMSAT Score. Note that many programmes (e.g. USyd, UniMelb) calculate the Overall score differently - they do not weight the Sciences section twice. Contact individual programmes for specific score requirements.

The GAMSAT may include a small number of questions which will not be scored. These questions are either used to calibrate the exam or were found to be either too ambiguous or too difficult to be counted or are trial questions which may be used in the future. So if you see a question that you think is off the wall, unanswerable or inappropriate for your level of knowledge, it could well be one of these questions so never panic! And of course, answer every question because guessing provides a 25% chance of being correct while not answering provides a 0% chance of being correct!

1.3.1 GAMSAT Scores in Different Countries

GAMSAT scores are interchangeable and can be used to apply to any university that requires the GAMSAT. You may sit the GAMSAT in the UK, Australia or Ireland to apply to universities in any of these countries. You must ensure that your scores have not expired if you are using a score from a previous sitting of the GAMSAT. Otherwise, you choose the GAMSAT score that you wish to submit for consideration for admissions.

Since there is no limit to the number of times you can sit the GAMSAT, you may even choose to sit the exam twice in one year. "Each year just under half of the questions in Sections 1 and 3 are new," according to *GAMSAT: A 10-year retrospective over-*

view, with detailed analysis of candidates' performance (BMC Med Educ. 2015; 15: 31; PMCID: PMC4351698). Despite the fact that over 50% of the multiple-choice questions are repeated, the study found a relatively small GAMSAT score increase (approx. 4/100, overall) with the first repeat, and little evidence of an upward trend thereafter. It seems clear that adequate preparation is more effective than constant repetition.

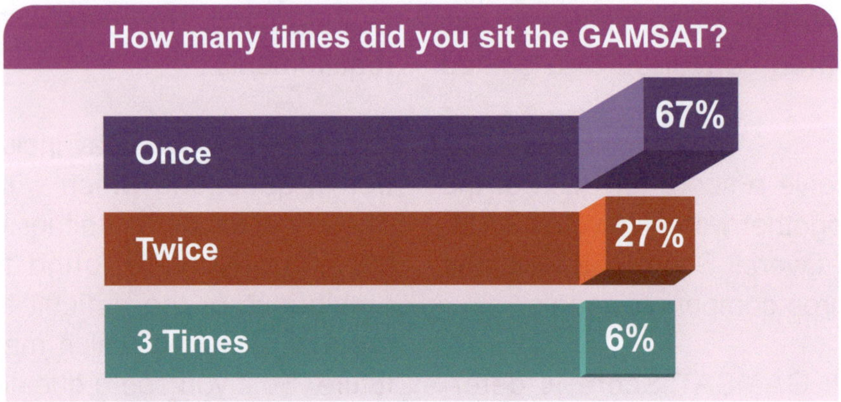

2010 Gold Standard GAMSAT survey at the University of Sydney (Usyd Medical Science Society), n>100, average reported GAMSAT score (most recent): 62.2. Our study seems consistent with the upward trend reported by ACER: 31% of the cohort had repeated the GAMSAT in 2005, up to 45% in 2014.

1.3.2 Average, Good and High GAMSAT Scores

Please keep in mind that the percentile rank indicates your test performance relative to all the students who sat the same test on the same day. It records the percentage of students whose scores were lower than yours.

Score	Percentile	Score
56-58	50th	average
61-63	75th	usually good*
73 or higher	98th	very high

*Please note, a "good" score may be good enough for admittance to one particular medical school but below the cutoff of another. Consult the websites of the medical institutions to which you intend to apply. Click on your national icon at the following webpage to get a summary of scores required at institutions near you: www.gamsat-prep.com/GAMSAT-scores.

An average GAMSAT score is often around 56-58 and a high GAMSAT score is over 63. Please keep in mind when evaluating the statistics provided and the graphic: this data is meant to give you a general idea of the process. The numbers can vary somewhat from one exam sitting to another. And as mentioned previously, you cannot replicate the scoring system at home since there is no formula provided to convert raw scores into official GAMSAT scores. Note that a score above 80 is very rare.

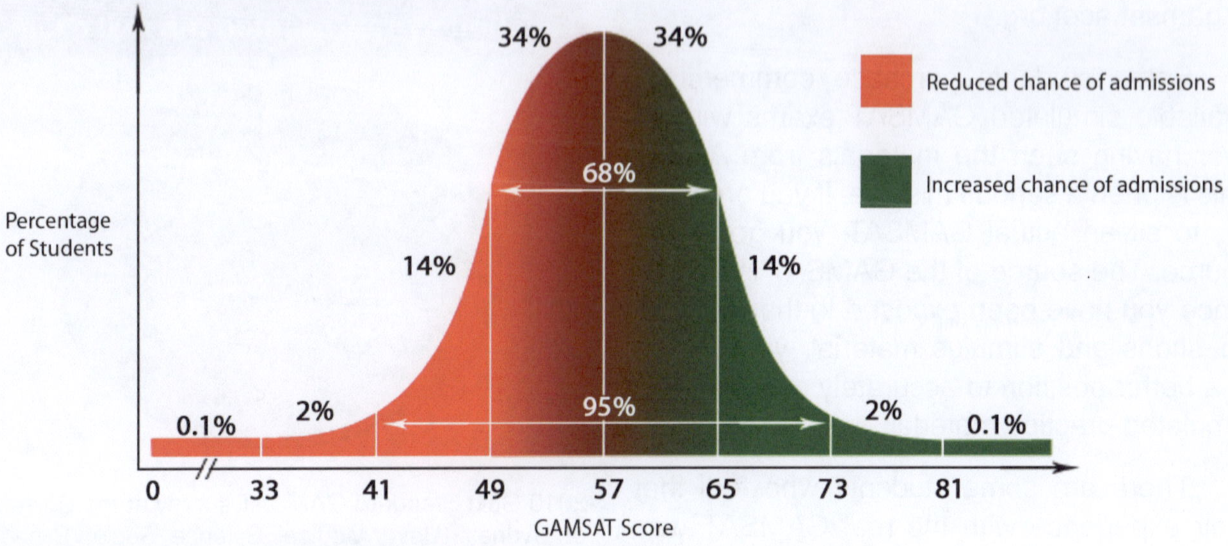

Figure 1: Typical Overall GAMSAT Score Distribution (Approx.)

1.3.3 When are the scores released?

GAMSAT is held twice a year, in March and September. GAMSAT results are released within 2 months of sitting the exam. Candidates are emailed login information to access their personal results report. Should there be any changes to the exam dates or any other modifications, get the up-to-date information online at gamsat.acer.org.

1.4 ACER

The GAMSAT has been developed by the Australian Council for Educational Research (ACER) with the Consortium of Graduate Medical Schools to help in the selection of students to graduate-entry programmes. ACER administers the GAMSAT and publishes several important sets of materials which are available on their website: i) GAMSAT Practice

Questions; ii) GAMSAT Sample Questions; and iii) GAMSAT Practice Test 1, GAMSAT Practice Test 2, and GAMSAT Practice Test 3, which are released operational full-length tests (pre-2020, paper version).

These materials can be obtained online at gamsat.acer.org.

Some students purchase commercially available simulated GAMSAT exams without ever having seen the materials from ACER. This is often a serious mistake. If you are looking to sit an actual GAMSAT, you go to the source. The source of the GAMSAT is ACER. Once you have been exposed to their style of questions and stimulus material, you will be in a better position to accurately assess other simulated practice material.

There are some students who feel that their experience with the real GAMSAT was not well represented by ACER's practice materials. Usually, this is not a problem with the materials; rather, it is a problem with the technique used in preparation. We will discuss this in detail in the next chapter.

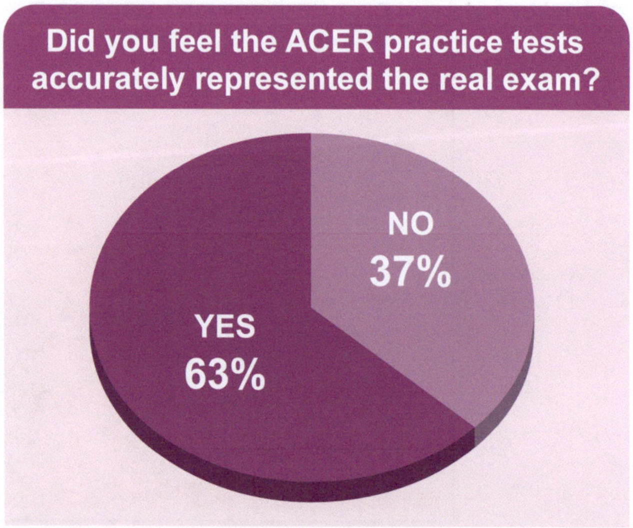

2010 Gold Standard GAMSAT survey at the University of Sydney (Usyd Medical Science Society), n>100, average reported GAMSAT score (most recent): 62.2.

1.5 Living a GAMSAT Life

Any discussion regarding the structure of the GAMSAT should end with a reminder of what the exam's structure means to you. Using your best reasoning skills with focus for an entire day is very challenging. Add to this the stress due to the importance of the exam, queues, nervous habits of other examinees, varying temperature/sounds/smells, etc., and you can quickly get a sense as to the unique nature of this exam.

We can give you the tools to get your mind ready. But, you must also get your body ready. For at least 2 weeks, every day prior to the real sitting of the exam, live your life like the exam's schedule. Wake up at the intended time, schedule similar meals, spend most of your waking hours intellectually engaged and, no naps! Ideally, your days would include practice tests followed by at least one full day to analyse the exam while taking very brief, top-level notes (*Gold Notes*). Your evenings could include exercise, hobbies and Gold Notes' revision.

THE RECIPE FOR GAMSAT SUCCESS

2.1 The Important Ingredients

- Time, Motivation
- gamsat-prep.com/free-GAMSAT-study-schedule
- Read from varied sources
- The Gold Standard (GS) GAMSAT YouTube videos
- A study of the 4 basic GAMSAT sciences

GAMSAT-specific Information

- The Masters Series GAMSAT textbooks
- *optional:* The Gold Standard GAMSAT videos, apps, tutorials or other online programs (GAMSAT-prep.com)
- *optional:* GS and/or ACER Essay Correction Service or GAMSAT University online.
- *optional*: YouTube Chemistry/Physics and/or History/Philosophy Crash Course, or Khan Academy
- *AVOID:* uni. textbooks (too much detail), upper-level courses for the purpose of improving GAMSAT scores

GAMSAT-specific Problems

- Free GS additional practice questions online
- The Gold Standard GAMSAT full-length practice test with the new digital format (GS-Free)
- Official ACER practice materials and full-length tests
- *optional:* Heaps of GAMSAT Sample Questions: 15 Full-length GAMSAT Practice Tests, 5 in the book and 10 online with the new digital format

If you could prepare all over again, what would you do differently?

Top 5 Responses

1. Study more
2. More practice essays
3. Newspapers, current events
4. More multiple-choice questions
5. More science revision

2010 Gold Standard GAMSAT survey at the University of Sydney (Usyd Medical Science Society), n>100, average reported GAMSAT score (most recent): 62.2.

2.2 The Proper Mix

1) Study regularly and start early. There is a lot of material to cover and you will need sufficient time to study it all adequately. Creating a study schedule is often effective. Consider going to gamsat-prep.com/free-GAMSAT-study-schedule and adapting our suggested, detailed study schedule to your own needs. Starting early will reduce your stress level in the weeks leading up to the exam and may make your studying easier. Depending on your English skills and the quality of your science background, a good rule of thumb is: 3-6 hours/day of study for 3-6 months. An avid reader with strong science-reasoning skills may require far less time, whereas someone with a non-science background (NSB) and little experience writing essays may require significantly more time.

2) Keep focused and enjoy the material you are learning. Forget all past negative learning experiences so you can open your mind to the information with a positive attitude. Given an open mind and some time to consider what you are learning, you will find most of the information tremendously interesting. Motivation can be derived from a sincere interest in learning and by keeping in mind your long-term goals.

3) Preparation for Non-sciences: Begin by reading the advice in this textbook as well as assessing The Gold Standard GAMSAT videos at gamsat-prep.com or on YouTube. Time yourself and practice, practice, practice with various resources for RHSS as needed at GAMSAT-prep.com and, of course, the ACER materials. You can also view free corrected WC essays: GAMSAT-prep.com/forum.

For RHSS, you should endeavour to understand each and every mistake you make as to ensure there will be improvement. For WC essays, you should have someone who has good-writing skills read, correct, and comment on your essays. And you also have the option of having your essays corrected, scored and returned to you with personal advice (GAMSAT-prep.com). ACER has introduced a program to automatically correct practice essays which you should seriously consider.

4) Preparation for Sciences: The Gold Standard is not associated with ACER in any way; however, our new Masters Series science books contain each and every topic that you are responsible for in the Biological and Physical Sciences, as evidenced by past testing patterns. Thus the most directed and efficient study plan is to begin by learning from - not memorising - the science sections in those textbooks. While doing your science survey, you should take notes specifically on topics that are marked Memorise or Understand on the first page of each chapter. Your notes, we call them Gold Notes (!!), should be very concise (no longer than one page per chapter). Every week, you should study from your Gold Notes at least a few times, especially as the real exam approaches.

As you are incorporating the information from the sciences, complete the Biological and Physical Sciences problems included in those books. This is the best way to more clearly define the depth of your understanding and to get you accustomed to the most challenging of the questions you can expect on the GAMSAT.

5) **Sit practice exams.** Ideally, you would finish your study of the sciences at least a month prior to your real exam date. Then each week you can sit 1-3 practice exams under simulated test conditions and thoroughly analyse each exam experience after completion. GAMSAT scores from practice exams should improve over time. Success depends on what you do between the first and the last exam. You can start with ACER's "GAMSAT Practice Questions" (it is free with registration and the easiest of their materials). Subsequently, you could continue with The Gold Standard (GS-Free, online), and then the Heaps practice exams, and finally, complete the practice materials from ACER.

You should sit practice exams as you would the actual test: within the expected time limits, similar time of day, etc. Sitting practice exams will increase your confidence and allow you to see what is expected of you. It will make you realise the constraints imposed by time limits in completing the entire test. It will also allow you to identify the areas in which you may be lacking.

Some students can answer all GAMSAT questions quite well if they only had more time. Thus you must time yourself during practice and monitor your time during the test. On average, you will have 1.6 minutes per question in RHSS and 2 minutes per question for Sciences. In other words, every 30 minutes, you should check to be sure that you have completed approximately 20 questions (RHSS) or 15 questions (Sciences). If not, then consider guessing on "time consuming questions" in order to catch up and, if you have time at the end, you return to properly evaluate the questions you skipped.

Set aside at least the equivalent of a full day to analyse the worked solutions to EVERY test question. Do NOT dismiss any wrong answer as a "stupid mistake." You made that error for a reason so you must work that out in your mind to reduce the risk that it occurs again. You can reduce your risk by testproofing answers (a technique first described in the Introduction to the GAMSAT video, GAMSAT-prep.com: spending 5-10 seconds being critical of your response). After your mock exam, you should consider the questions below.

1. Why did you get the question wrong (or correct)?
2. What question-type or passage-type gives you repeated difficulty?
3. What is your mindset when facing a particular passage?
4. Did you monitor your time during the test?
5. Are most of your errors at the beginning or the end of the test?
6. Did you eliminate answer choices when you could and actually cross them out on your scratch paper?
7. For Humanities and Social Sciences (RHSS), what was the author's mindset and main idea for each passage?
8. Was your main problem a lack of content revision or a lack of practice?
9. In which specific science-content areas do you need improvement?
10. Have you designed a study schedule to address your weaknesses?

6) **Big on concepts, small on memorisation:** Remember that the GAMSAT will primarily test your understanding of concepts. The GAMSAT is not designed to measure your ability to memorise tons of scientific facts and trivia, but both your knowledge and understanding of concepts are critical.

Evidently, some material in the Masters Series textbooks must be memorised; for example, some very basic science equations (i.e. weight W = mg, Ohm's Law, Newton's Second Law, etc.), rules of logarithms, trigonometric functions, the phases in mitosis and meiosis, naming organic compounds, and other basic science facts. Based on past-testing patterns, we will guide you. Nonetheless, for the most part, your objective should be to try to understand, rather than memorise the biology, physics and chemistry material you will be studying. This may appear vague now, but as you immerse yourself in the science chapters and practice material, you will more clearly understand what is expected of you.

7) **Relax once in a while!** While the GAMSAT requires a lot of preparation, you should not forsake all your other activities to study. Try to keep exercising, maintain a social life and engage in activities that you enjoy. If you balance work with stress-reducing experiences, you will study more effectively overall.

2.3 It's GAMSAT Time!

1) On the night before the exam, try to get a good night's sleep. The GAMSAT is physically draining and it is in your best interest to be well rested when you sit the exam.

2) Avoid last minute cramming. On the morning of the exam, do not begin studying ad hoc. You will not learn anything effectively, and noticing something you do not know or will not remember might reduce your confidence and lower your score unnecessarily. Just get up, eat a good breakfast, consult your Gold Notes (the top-level information that you personally compiled) and go sit the exam.

3) Eat breakfast! It will make it possible for you to have the food energy needed to go through the first two parts of the exam.

4) Pack a light lunch. Avoid greasy food that may make you drowsy. You do not want to sleep during Sciences! Avoid sugar-packed snacks as they may cause a 'sugar low' eventually and also make you drowsy. The choices you make regarding your exam-day diet, including a judicious use of caffeine, should be informed by your GAMSAT 'prep' in the weeks prior to your real exam. If you do not already know what is best, experiment early!

5) Make sure you answer all the questions! You do not get penalised for incorrect answers, so always choose something even if you have to guess. If you run out of time, pick a letter and use it to answer all the remaining questions. ACER performs statistical analyses on every test so no one letter will

give you an unfair advantage so just choose your "lucky" letter and move on!

6) Pace yourself. Do not get bogged down trying to answer a difficult question. If the question is very difficult, write the question number on your scratch paper, guess, move on to the next question and return later if time is remaining.

7) Remember that some of the questions may be thrown out as inappropriate, used solely to calibrate the test or trial questions. If you find that you cannot answer some of the questions, do not despair. It is possible they could be questions used for these purposes.

8) Do not let others psyche you out! Some people will be saying, between exam sections, 'It went great. What a joke!' Ignore them. Often these types may just be trying to boost their own confidence or to make themselves look good in front of their friends. Just focus on what you have to do and tune out the other examinees.

9) Do not study at lunch. You need the time to recuperate and rest. Eat, avoid the people discussing the test sections and relax! At most, you can revise your Gold Notes.

10) Before reading the "stimulus material" of the problem (the passage, article, etc.), some students find it more efficient to quickly read the questions first. In this way, as soon as you read something in the stimulus material which brings to mind a question you have read, you can answer immediately (this is especially helpful for Humanities and Social Sciences, RHSS). Otherwise, if you read the text first and then the questions, you may end up wasting time searching through the text for answers.

11) Read the text and questions carefully! Often students leave out a word or two while reading, which can completely change the sense of the problem. Pay special attention to words in italics, CAPS, bolded, or underlined. Briefly note on your scratch paper anything you believe might be very important in the passage.

12) You will be selecting an answer by clicking one of four radio buttons next to the answer options. You must be both diligent and careful because you will not be given extra time to either check it or fill it in later.

13) If you are running out of time, just complete the questions. In other words, only read the part of the passage which your question specifically requires in order for you to get the correct answer.

14) Expel any relevant equation onto your scratch paper! Even if the question is of a theoretical nature, sometimes equations contain the answers and they are much more objective than the reasoning of a nervous pre-medical student! In physics, it is often helpful to draw a picture or diagram. Arrows are valuable in representing vectors.

15) Consider having the following on test day: layers of clothes so that you are ready for too much heat or an overzealous air-conditioning unit.

16) Solving the problem may involve algebraic manipulation of equations and/or numerical calculations. Be sure that you know what all the variables in the equation stand for and that you are using the equation in the appropriate circumstance.

In chemistry and physics, the use of **dimensional analysis** will help you keep track of units and solve some problems where you might have forgotten the relevant equations (we will discuss this topic rigorously in Masters Series Maths, Chapter 2). Dimensional analysis relies on the manipulation of units and is the source of many easy GAMSAT marks every year. For example, if you are asked for the energy involved in maintaining a 60-watt bulb lit for two minutes you can pull out the appropriate equations or: **(i)** recognise that your objective (unknown = energy) is in joules; **(ii)** recall that a watt is a joule per second; **(iii)** convert minutes into seconds. {note that minutes and seconds cancel leaving joules as an answer}

$$60 \frac{\text{joules}}{\text{second}} \times 2 \text{ minutes} \times 60 \frac{\text{seconds}}{\text{minute}}$$

$$= 7200 \text{ joules or } 7.2 \text{ kilojoules}$$

17) The final step in problem-solving is to ask yourself: *is my answer reasonable*? For example, if you would have done the preceding problem and your answer was 7200 kilojoules, intuitively, this should strike you as an exorbitant amount of energy for an everyday light bulb to remain lit for two minutes! It would then be of value to recheck your calculations. {*'intuition' in science is often learned through the experience of doing many problems; if you do not have a science background, do not worry about the preceding points, we will be exploring dimensional analysis throughout the Masters Series Biological Sciences and Physical Sciences textbooks including the chapter practice questions.*}

18) Whenever doing calculations, the following will increase your speed: **(i)** manipulate variables but plug in values only when necessary; **(ii)** avoid decimals, use fractions wherever possible; **(iii)** square roots or cube roots can be converted to the power (*exponent*) of 1/2 or 1/3, respectively; **(iv)** before calculating, check to see if the possible answers are sufficiently far apart such that your values can be approximated (i.e. $19.2 \approx 20$, $185 \approx 200$). Since 2012, calculators ceased being permitted for the GAMSAT. We added over 150 pages of GAMSAT Maths to help you become quick and efficient with your calculations.

19) Are you great in biology and organic chemistry but weak in the physical sciences? Since biology and organic chemistry represent more than 1/2 your science score, you should attack those problems from the outset to ensure that you have fully benefitted from your strengths. Now you can go back and complete the physics and general chemistry. This is just an example of 'examsmanship': managing the test to maximise your performance (we will discuss 'examsmanship' again in the context of RHSS in section 3.2.3).

20) Learn to relax or at least you must learn to manage your anxiety. Channel that extra energy into acute awareness of the information being presented to you. If you have a history of anxiety during exams to the extent that you feel that it affected your score, then you should start learning relaxation techniques now. You can search online regarding various methods such as visualisation, mindfulness exercises, deep breathing and other techniques that can be used during the exam if needed.

GAMSAT-Prep.com

REASONING IN HUMANITIES AND SOCIAL SCIENCES

PREPARATION FOR RHSS

3.1 Overview

GAMSAT Humanities and Social Sciences (officially, Reasoning in Humanities and Social Sciences, or RHSS) is, for many applicants, the most difficult section to do well. This can be explained by the absence of an overall set of facts to study in order to prepare. Due to the lack of an official list of test content, some applicants either struggle or simply neglect to prepare for this section.

While the best preparation is regular reading from a variety of sources throughout your high school (*secondary school*) and undergraduate studies, it is also possible to improve your ability to do well in this section as you approach the test date. You should not neglect to prepare for this section as it accounts for one of your final GAMSAT numerical scores!

You are provided with 100 minutes to answer 62 questions (i.e., the digital GAMSAT timing since 2022; before 2020: 100 minutes for 75 questions). This section consists of a number of "Units" where each Unit presents stimulus material and a number of multiple-choice questions (4 options per question).

The stimulus material in RHSS can be anything from a poem, a cartoon, an extract from a play, novel, song, instructional manual or magazine. Essentially anything that involves words or symbols and thinking is fair game. There is no specific presumed knowledge required to answer any of the questions.

Reasoning, analysis, timing and pacing are all key components to success.

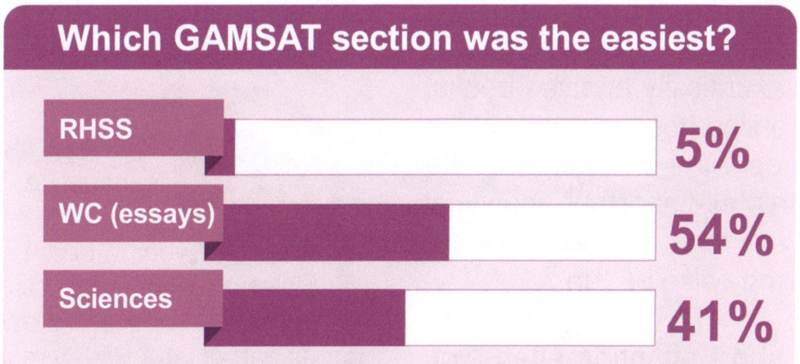

2010 Gold Standard GAMSAT survey at the University of Sydney, n>100, <5% with a non-science background; average reported GAMSAT score (most recent): 62.2.

3.2 How to Prepare for GAMSAT Humanities and Social Sciences

3.2.1 One Year or More Before the GAMSAT

Medium-level Importance

Read! Be known as a "voracious reader"! In the real exam, you will be presented with varying types of texts and language styles that range from literary, academic, instructional to numerical data and visual representations. You may encounter a few passages discussing unfamiliar topics or using convoluted language - or both! Additionally, you will have to deal with time pressure. Overcoming GAMSAT Humanities and Social Sciences (RHSS), therefore, requires two interdependent reading skills: speed and comprehension.

Reading is fundamentally about language comprehension. If you aim to improve your reading speed, the best solution would be to read a repertoire of diverse materials in order to expand your vocabulary and in effect, increase your comprehension. Develop a "love" for reading. Read any novel that interests you. Read editorials from national, international and local newspapers (among your options: the reference section of the library or online).

Develop ways to critically analyse books: Consider joining an online book club or even a book club where people meet in person! The point is to develop this all-important analytical GAMSAT skill in an environment that is conducive to learning and may also be fun.

If you have a short attention span, you can start with Ted.com. You will have powerful, easy-to-digest lectures on a great range of topics. Many of the videos will further develop your skills for learning new information and exercising the use of language through analogies, research, and stories spanning the globe as well as time. For the purpose of improving your language comprehension skills for RHSS, choose Ted.com topics that involve controversies related to social values and ethical dilemmas in the practice of medicine and health care.

Ted.com is a free website. We will always update further suggestions on GAMSAT-prep.com which you can find by clicking on FREE GAMSAT in the top menu. Please do note that RHSS is not a test about pre-existing knowledge but about reasoning based on the given stimulus. Hence you should go through these materials with the purpose of identifying the main ideas, arguments, intents of the speakers or writers, any implicit meanings in the text, as well as expanding your vocabulary.

> **!** Our list is neither definitive nor exhaustive. These are merely suggestions to help develop your familiarity with the language styles and the typical pieces used in RHSS passages. You are free to add other selections as part of your RHSS reading library.

Ideally, you should spend an hour and a half daily reading a variety of written and visual pieces. Otherwise, you should endeavour to read at least once per week, for 1-3 hours, any of the following (many of which are available in a university library or online):

- **Articles from Medical Journals**

  Many medical journals publish articles that are accessible online free of charge. Access to the full texts may require registration for a free user account. Look for articles on medical ethics, scientific studies that include graphs, tables and figures, sections on medicine and the arts, poetry, narratives and opinions from the doctors' as well as the patients' perspectives. The following are some of the most popular medical journals:

  PubMed Central is a free access repository of scholarly articles published in the biomedical and life sciences journal literature at the U.S. National Institutes of Health's National Library of Medicine.

  The Medical Journal of Australia has made all their MJA research articles published since 2002 open access and available free of charge online.

  The BMJ (formerly the British Medical Journal) is an international peer-reviewed medical journal published by the BMJ Publishing Group Ltd, which is a wholly-owned subsidiary of the British Medical Association. It provides full access to journal articles in its online archive.

  Irish Medical Journal is a free access general medical journal published by the Irish Medical Organisation, which features full-text scientific research, review articles, updates and reflections on contemporary clinical practices.

  The Lancet Journals are produced by Elsevier Ltd and feature selected free full-text research articles and review content.

  JAMA (Journal of the American Medical Association) is a peer-reviewed medical journal published by the American Medical Association with several free access texts covering original research, reviews, and editorials on various aspects of the biomedical sciences.

- **Creative Nonfiction**

  This genre includes essays, memoirs, autobiographies, biographies, travel writing, history, cultural studies and nature writing with topics that span just about everything under the sun. The following selections will likely provide a good overview of typical subjects and writing styles found in some RHSS Units.

  - Charles Darwin (1859). *On the Origin of Species*
  - Joan Didion (2006). *We Tell Ourselves Stories in Order to Live: Collected Nonfiction*
  - Patrick Leigh Fermor (1977). *A Time of Gifts*
  - Michel Foucault (1975). *Discipline and Punish*
  - Sigmund Freud (1899). *The Interpretation of Dreams*
  - Stephen Jay Gould (1977). *Ever Since Darwin: Reflections in Natural History*

- Catherine Hamlin *(2005). The Hospital by the River*
- Thomas Kuhn (1962). *The Structure of Scientific Revolutions*
- V. S. Naipaul (1999). *Between Father and Son: Family Letters*
- George Orwell (1961). *Collected Essays*
- Joseph Sacco (1989). *Morphine, Ice Cream, Tears: Tales of a City Hospital*
- Susan Sontag (1966). *Against Interpretation and Other Essays*
- Lionel Trilling (1950). *The Liberal Imagination: Essays on Literature and Society*
- Abraham Verghese (1994). *My Own Country: A Doctor's Story*
- Ludwig Wittgenstein (1953). *Philosophical Investigations*
- Virginia Woolf (1929). *A Room of One's Own*

Editorials and News Articles

The 'Opinions' section of reputable national newspapers tends to be argumentative, which is typical of RHSS passages. Newspaper cartoons also use a style of humour and presentation that is fair game for the GAMSAT. Occasionally, news reports come with graphs and tables, which could help expose you to various types of graphical data. All of these make good sources for developing the reading speed and comprehension necessary for Humanities and Social Sciences.

- The Economist
- The Australian
- The Guardian
- The Irish Independent
- The New Yorker
- The Telegraph

Performing a reanalysis of the novels, plays, and poems you encountered in Year 12 - or A Level - could help prepare you to tackle exam content featuring excerpts from literary works. Nevertheless, the following lists should be able to get you started with your literary reading. As a reminder, these are merely suggested titles and should not be taken as an official guide.

Novels

- Any Jane Austen novel
- Julian Barnes (1980). *Metroland*
- Karel Čapek (1936). *War With The Newts (a.k.a. War With The Salamanders)*
- Charles Dickens (1861). *Great Expectations*
- George Eliot (1871). *Middlemarch*
- F. Scott Fitzgerald (1922). *The Beautiful and Damned*
- Charlotte Perkins Gilman (1892). *The Yellow Wallpaper*

- Henry James (1881). *Portrait of a Lady*
- CS Lewis *(1942). The Screwtape Letters*
- Gabriel García Márquez (1967). *One Hundred Years of Solitude*
- Ian McEwan (1997). *Enduring Love*
- Patrick O'Brian (1972). *Post Captain*
- Brian O'Nolan (1939). *At Swim-Two-Birds*
- George Orwell (1949). *Nineteen Eighty-Four*
- Boris Pasternak (1957). *Doctor Zhivago*
- Leo Tolstoy (1869). *War and Peace*

- **Plays**
  - Euripides (412 BC). *Andromeda*
  - Christopher Marlowe (1592). *Dr Faustus*
  - William Shakespeare (1604). *Othello*
  - Sophocles (441 BC). *Antigone*
- **Poetry**
  - Any anthology book of poetry
  - Poems written by medical practitioners and medical students
  - Poems with subjects on medicine, science or in hospital settings
  - Some notable poets whose pieces make interesting reading for your RHSS preparation are Dannie Abse, George Barker, Elizabeth Bishop, Emily Dickinson, Gwen Harwood, A. D. Hope, Elizabeth Jennings, John Keats, Philip Larkin, Sylvia Plath, William Shakespeare, Walt Whitman, and Virginia Woolf.

Again, your main goal in reading these materials is to increase your comprehension by becoming accustomed to the highly diverse themes and writing styles of RHSS passages. Oftentimes, the difficulty of a specific Unit is subjective to an examinee. Someone who is not used to reading poetry and classic novels, for example, or dense articles from medical journals would find these passages very challenging to understand because of limited exposure to such topics. Therefore, while no prior knowledge is required to answer any of the questions, your exposure to concepts involving creativity, culture, literature, current affairs, political cartoons and more will have a significant impact on your performance in RHSS and even in GAMSAT Written Communication (essays). The added benefit - which you may only appreciate later - will be your improved performance in the medical school interviews and possibly even less obvious at the moment - an increased well-roundedness.

In addition, active reading tends to improve comprehension and speed, so be sure that when you are reading, especially opinion pieces, you are continually asking questions:

1) How would you summarise or simplify what is being presented?
2) What are the main points of the author?

3) What types of evidence does the author employ to support a point?

4) How would you describe the author's attitude to the topic?

The following reading techniques may also prove helpful:

1. Skimming

This is a technique for spotting clues within the text itself. You run your eyes quickly through the content for an overview of what to expect in the material, occasionally slowing down on salient parts. As you skim over the words and the paragraphs, figure out which parts are essential and which are not. Using this technique will allow you to detect parts where you need to dedicate some attention for a better understanding of the material.

2. Paraphrasing

This reading technique is highly applicable to selections from the humanities and any text that demand inference. In order to test your general understanding of the reading material, restate the main idea of each relevant paragraph. By the end of the article, you will have a clearer outline of the author's central point. Taking the whole by its smaller parts is less overwhelming than having to swallow everything in a single glance.

3. Visualising

This technique usually works best with literary pieces such as poetry and novels. You mentally picture the colours and movements described in the different lines in order to capture the setting, the qualities and motives of a character, or the sentiment that the author wishes to express.

The new, digital GAMSAT RHSS typically consists of 9 to 12 units

- **1-2** units of philosophical texts
- **1-3** units of cartoons
- **1-3** units of excerpts from novels or plays
- **1-3** units of a single poem or a group of poems
- **1-3** units of tables and diagrams
- **3** or more units of creative nonfiction

3.2.2 One Year or Less Before the GAMSAT

Read RHSS 3.2.1 one more time! Even at this point in your preparation, being a voracious reader - with all that it entails - should remain your goal. This time, however, aim to develop a reading speed of at least 350 words per minute and an 80% comprehension rate. If you would like to check your current reading efficiency level, you may attempt the short test in RHSS 3.7.4.

It is important to note that your reading speed will likely fluctuate depending on the type of material you're perusing. For example, you might find that you can read and understand articles from newspapers much faster than those from medical journals; and yet, you have to re-read poems and classic novels several times before you can fully comprehend them. This is why familiarity with different types of texts is quite important. Besides improving your language comprehension, it allows you to gauge your timing and adjust your strategy for each type of passage in RHSS. (Please *see* RHSS 3.2.3 for further discussion on this point.)

Contextual reading is another essential skill that you will need to develop for Section I, especially because almost 80% of the total units will have at least one question asking for the meaning of a word or its nuances in the passage's context. With contextual reading, you will learn how to make a logical guess about the meaning of an unfamiliar word based on the other words and phrases found within the immediate sentences in the paragraph. Writers themselves use this technique to make lucid points. Several cues easily offer probable definitions to uncommon terms:

1) Examples

Cue words: includes, consists of, such as

Equine *animals, such as horses and zebras, have long been used not only to aid in man's work but also to assist in therapy.*

Using the example clue (the use of "such as"), the word equine means:

A. *mammal.*
B. *reptile.*
C. *horse group.*
D. *dog.*

2) Synonyms

Cue words: is similar to, just as, also means

Calling my cousin an "eccentric weirdo" is ***tautologous****! It is similar to telling a ghost that he is dead twice.*

Medium-level Importance

The cue word "is similar to" indicates that tautologous means:

A. *repetitive.*
B. *alien.*
C. *scary.*
D. *ridiculous.*

3) Antonyms and Contrasts

Cue words: unlike, contrary to/in contrast, on the other hand, as opposed to

*Contrary to the playwright's **euphemisms** about the King's corrupt leadership, the merchant was quite direct in criticising the latter's injustices.*

Based on the contrasting descriptions used in the sentence, the word euphemism refers to:

A. *corruption.*
B. *indirect speech.*
C. *criticism.*
D. *politics.*

Answers

1. C
2. A
3. B

4) Sense of the sentence

Oftentimes, you only need to observe how the words or phrases relate within the sentence in order to fairly conclude what the difficult word means. Take careful note of the descriptions in the paragraph. Use your logic to determine the most probable meaning of a newly-encountered term.

*March 21, 1894 marks a rare series of **syzygies** in the history of astronomical events. A few hours before Mercury transits the sun as seen from Venus, a partial lunar eclipse is witnessed from Earth. From Saturn, both Mercury and Venus could be seen simultaneously transiting the sun. Such planetary spectacles can also be observed by the naked human eye during full moons and new moons as the sun, our planet Earth, and the moon periodically align.*

Based on the context of the discussion in the paragraph, the closest meaning of syzygies could be:

A. *planetary collisions.*
B. *lunar eclipses.*
C. *planetary alignments.*
D. *historical changes.*

Answer

Descriptions in the paragraph mention "lunar eclipse," "Mercury transits the sun" and "the sun, our planet Earth, and the moon periodically align." These should serve as primary clues in determining a general definition of syzygies.

(D) Historical changes is obviously the least likely option. (A) Planetary collisions may sound related; however, nothing in the paragraph indicates a collision of the planets. This should now narrow down your choice between (B) lunar eclipses and (C) planetary alignments. Now common knowledge tells us that a lunar eclipse occurs when three celestial bodies such as the sun, the moon and the Earth align. On the other hand, a full moon or a new moon does not necessarily result in a lunar eclipse. This makes C the more logical answer!

Medium-level Importance

5) Root Words, Prefixes, and Suffixes

Certain root words and word parts carry specific meanings. Being acquainted with these, combined with the other clues discussed earlier, helps you figure out the most probable meaning of an unfamiliar word.

If you have less than 6 months preparation time left, you should still try to read many of the selections in our suggested list. However, another approach that might improve your efficiency in tackling RHSS units exploring creative nonfiction, novels and plays would be to read the synopsis of famous works on reputable 'Study Guide' websites such as SparkNotes.com and CliffsNotes.com. Again, your main objective in adopting this approach is to acquaint yourself with the plot, theme, characters, and symbolisms of as many literary pieces as possible. Attempt the chapter or study quizzes provided by these websites in order to increase your comprehension.

Besides reading, you need to practice. The best strategy is to take ACER's GAMSAT Practice Questions, aka the red booklet (it is not a full-length test), and sit RHSS as a timed exam and then study from your mistakes. This should be done as soon as you commence your preparation. The ACER booklets are the closest that you will get to the real exam.

Using one of the shorter practice tests as a baseline of your test performance under timed conditions will help you understand what is expected. Take note of the type of passages and questions that give you the most difficulty (e.g., poetry, cartoon, prose, commentaries). This will enable you to slowly build on your weaknesses and target particular problem areas.

The full-length ACER practice exams should be completed later in the preparation process to further measure your performance while providing enough time to continually address your weaknesses.

If you performed well and understood the source of your errors then you will only require ACER and the Gold Standard (GS) GAMSATs in order to complete your preparation for RHSS.

If, on the other hand, you struggled in the test or struggled to understand your mistakes then you may need additional work on strategies, practice or, as mentioned previously, a formal course with or without credit. An optional RHSS GAMSAT program can be found at GAMSAT-prep.com, as well as 5 full-length GS GAMSAT practice tests and the GAMSAT Heaps book featuring an unprecedented 15 full-length mock tests.

Practice Problems
• ACER materials
• GS books and online

Practice Exams
• ACER materials
• GS books and online
• 5 GS Online GAMSAT Practice Tests
• GAMSAT Heaps: 15 Full-length Practice Tests for the GAMSAT (this includes GS tests)

High-level Importance

3.2.3 Exam Strategies

Candidates have aced this section using different strategies. There is no "one size fits all" strategy to obtain a great score. The key is to be able to start early with your preparation so you can identify which strategy specifically works for you. A systematic approach with clear strategies – a 'game plan' – is vital in achieving an excellent RHSS score.

Ideally, you should make a concerted effort to try the various strategies that we will discuss in this section during separate timed practice tests. Then you can compare the various scores which you have obtained. This will help you narrow down the specific strategies which give you your optimal performance. From that point onward, you should remain consistent.

• Time Management Strategies

One of your main aims in sitting timed practice exams is to gradually reach a speed where you have at least 10 minutes to spare. If you have time in the end, you can return to properly evaluate the questions you skipped or guessed. Start adopting the following time management strategies early in your preparation to master your exam speed.

1) Maximise the Reading Time

Technically, reading time is a legacy issue from the 'old' paper GAMSAT when students were forbidden to answer questions during that period. The new digital GAMSAT permits you to answer questions as soon as the timer starts so there is no formal reading time. However, the concept of quickly identifying various types of passages to estimate and adjust your speed according to the difficulty level of the texts, or by seeking your favourite question type, like poetry or drama, and writing the question numbers on your scratch paper (provided by the test centre), remain effective strategies.

2) 'Examsmanship'

Play to your strengths. The following can be quite effective for both RHSS and Written Communication (essays):

Now that you have identified the locations of your favourite content, begin answering those questions. Although out of sequence, answer all the question types that you are most comfortable with and then go back to answer the rest of the questions. Fill in the digital radio buttons as you go along but be very diligent to ensure that you are always answering the correct question. As always, keep an eye on the time. By playing to your strengths, you can maximise your score.

3) Pace Yourself

A major problem in this section is that test takers run out of time. Read at a reasonable speed. You want to read carefully but quickly. You will have just over 1.5 minutes per question for the new, digital GAMSAT RHSS. Every 30 minutes, you should check the clock/timer to be sure that you have completed approximately 20 questions. By maintaining that pace, you will have about 7 minutes left at the end to double-check challenging questions.

Of course, you can judge time in any way you want (20, 25, 30-minute intervals, etc.). But decide on a system when you are practising then stick to that system on exam day.

You should still prepare for any contingency in the actual sitting. After all, no one knows what specific topics and questions will appear on exam day. If you have not completed the desired number of questions in the interval that you have set for yourself, then you consistently guess on time-consuming questions in order to catch up; and if you have time in the end, you return to properly evaluate the questions you skipped or marked.

- **Exam Reading Strategies**

As much as possible, refrain from skimming through the stimulus material. Ideally, you only want to read through once in order to answer the questions correctly. If you deliberately focus on locating main ideas and important details, your speed and comprehension usually increase. This enables you to finish in the allotted time. Rereading lines in the passage interrupts the flow of comprehension and will only slow you down. Of course, referring back to material that you annotated is not the same as having to re-read a passage because you read too quickly the first time.

The following are only a few of the proven methods employed by past candidates. They vary in their attack of the passages and questions. The most logical means to find out which strategy - or which combination of strategies - would augment your test-taking skills is to practice. The more you practice, the more you are inclined to be comfortable with a particular strategy and to modify or even create a new technique to suit your own strengths or weaknesses.

1) Questions First, Passage Once

Some candidates like to get a glimpse of the questions prior to reading the text. Others read the questions but not the answer choices yet. Then they read the passage and answer questions as they read the information (usu. the questions are placed in the same order as you would find the answers in the passage). The point of doing this is to survey the kind of reading technique that will work best in attacking the passage and which other strategy to employ.

You may find it more efficient to work in this manner. Try one of the practice exams using this strategy and if you find it easier to answer the questions correctly, you should use the same method on the actual GAMSAT.

2) Passage First, Questions Next

Some examinees prefer to carefully read the passage once while noting the key details. You can take brief notes of the major ideas and concepts in each paragraph along with their keywords. You can use boxes or circles to categorise the important details and then, make meaningful connections between the main concepts and their supporting information by using arrows. This is also called "mapping".

This strategy allows you to mark significant information in specific paragraphs so that they are easier to locate when answering relevant questions later. At the same time, you can see where the discussion is going as you construct each part of the "map". Ideally, you should be able to make a reasonable conclusion of the author's central thesis once you complete the "map".

3) Read the Opening and Closing Paragraphs

In many cases, you would need to combine one or two of the preceding approaches in dealing with the passages. Going over the first and last paragraphs of a passage gives you a "bracket" to work within. Once you get an initial feel of the passage, you can decide on the appropriate strategy that will speed up your performance during the exam.

4) Read Carefully and Annotate

The test is yours, interact with the exam. Experiment with taking very brief notes using your scratch paper. For 'process of elimination' questions, consider writing the question number and answer choices (just the letters) to strikeout as you move towards the correct answer. Doing so keeps your attention from wandering and helps you to read actively so that later, you can find keywords or points without having to search aimlessly.

5) Identifying the Main Ideas

Many of the Units will have questions that require you to determine the central idea of the passage and distinguish opposing arguments. Therefore, always try to identify the main points of each paragraph, the idea behind the text and the structure of the passage as you read. Doing this will make it easier for you to answer the questions.

Some students find it helpful to do the following: just before you read from each Unit, imagine someone young that you know - for example, a younger brother, sister, cousin, etc. Imagine that once you finish reading the stimulus material, you will have to explain it to them in words that they understand. Keep that imagery during your evaluation of the material so you have a heightened sense of awareness and responsibility for what you are reading.

6) "Edutainment"

We have already established that reading diverse material in the period leading up to the exam will be useful since the stimulus material will be from a variety of sources. Use this reality to help you create a mindset that, in the exam, you are prepared for "edutainment".

You are ready to learn interesting, vibrant material which sometimes borders on a form of entertainment (novels, poems, cartoons, some articles, etc.). After completing a Unit, look forward to what you can learn and discover in the next Unit. Having properly prepared and then to sit the exam with the right attitude will give you an edge.

3.2.4 Question and Answer Techniques

Understanding the "science" of answering multiple-choice questions is another vital skill in dealing with not only the Reasoning in Humanities and Social Sciences section, but also with the GAMSAT exam as a whole. The following are general techniques used in answering test questions.

1) **Process of Elimination (PoE):** cross out any answers that are obviously wrong. Oftentimes, after crossing out clearly wrong answers, you will find yourself in a dilemma between two closely similar options. In this case, you should choose the more encompassing answer. For instance, if you cannot discriminate between options A and B, ask yourself: Does A include and speak for B? Does B include or speak for A? Choose the option that incorporates the idea of the other.

2) **Beware of the Extreme:** words such as always, never, perfect, totally, and completely are often (but not always) clues that the answer choice is incorrect.

3) **Comfortable Words:** moderate words such as normally, often, at times, and ordinarily are often included in answer choices that are correct.

4) **Mean Statements:** mean or politically incorrect statements are highly unlikely to be included in a correct answer choice. For example, if you see any of the following statements in an answer choice, you can pretty much guarantee that it is not the correct answer:

   Parents should abuse their children.
   Poor people are lazy.
   Religion is socially destructive.
   Torture is usually necessary.

5) **Never lose sight of the question:** by the time students read answer choices C and D, some have forgotten the question and are simply looking for "true" sounding statements; you can then fall into the next trap: choosing an option, which presents a statement that may be true but does not answer the question.

   True but False and False but True: for example,

   Answer Choice D: Most people are of average height. → This is a true statement.

   However, the question was: What is the weight of most people?

   Therefore, the true statement becomes the incorrect answer!
   Continually check the question and check or cross out right and wrong answers.

High-level Importance

6) **Be on the lookout for qualifiers such as NOT:** these may or may not be emphasised in the question stem or the options. They can also come in the form of double negatives in an attempt to confound you.

7) **Verbatim Statements:** a common decoy in most timed multiple-choice exams is presenting options with literal and direct quotes from the stimulus material. This is frequently an incorrect choice because of the context of the actual question.

SPOILER ALERT

Gold Standard has cross-referenced the content in this chapter to examples from ACER's official GAMSAT practice materials (note that only ACER sells their eBooks brand new). It is for you to decide when you want to explore these questions since you may want to preserve some of ACER's materials for timed mock-exam practice.

Number	1	2	3	4	5
Title	GAMSAT Practice Questions	GAMSAT Sample Questions	GAMSAT Practice Test 1	GAMSAT Practice Test 2	GAMSAT Practice Test 3

Examples – Articles from Medical Journals Q27-32 of 1, Q50-54 and Q55-57 of 5; Creative Nonfiction Q1-6 of 2, Q1-5 of 5; Editorials and News Articles Q18-22 of 3; Novels Q7-10 of 4, Q25-28 and Q41-45 of 5; Plays Q33-35 of 2; Poetry Q22-26 of 1 and Q62-64 of 3; Contextual Meaning Q2, Q19 and Q33 of 1; Q4 of 2; Q1 and Q6 of 3, Q44 of 4; Q36 of 5. Note that "Q" is followed by the question number, and, for example, "of 1" refers to booklet number 1 in the table above. Also note that your gamsat-prep.com Masters Series online account has direct links to the step-by-step worked solutions for all of ACER's science practice questions (the solutions can also be found in the Gold Standard GAMSAT YouTube Channel). The 15 full-length HEAPS GAMSAT practice tests (by Gold Standard) include exams that contain specific cross-references to this chapter within the worked solutions.

Chapter Checklist

- ☐ Access your free online account at www.gamsat-prep.com/gamsat-humanities-and-social-sciences to view answers and worked solutions for the 3 practice tests at the back of this book, as well as to access Humanities and Social Sciences discussion boards for any questions or comments that you may have about this book.
- ☐ Complete a maximum of 1 page of notes using symbols/abbreviations to represent the content in the foregoing section. These are your Gold Notes.
- ☐ Consider your options based on your optimal way of learning:
  - ☐ Create your own, tangible study cards or try the free app: Anki.
  - ☐ Record your voice reading your Gold Notes onto your smartphone (memos or audio files) and listen during exercise, transportation, etc.
  - ☐ Consider reading at least 1 source material every day (e.g., poems of a single author, a synopsis of a novel, an article from a scientific journal that caught your interest, etc.). Note down the main idea or ideas of the piece on your scratch paper. Determine or surmise the author's sentiment or purpose for writing the material.
- ☐ Schedule your full-length GAMSAT practice tests: ACER and/or HEAPS exams. Schedule one full day to complete a practice test and 1-2 days for a thorough assessment of worked solutions while adding to your abbreviated Gold Notes.
- ☐ Schedule and/or evaluate stress reduction techniques such as regular exercise (sports), yoga, meditation and/or mindfulness exercises (*see* YouTube for suggestions).

3.3 Style of Questions

i) **Knowledge:** Simply put, you will not be asked questions based on prior knowledge. The very simplest of GAM-SAT questions may ask you to recall infor-mation from a passage; however, this is rare. Most questions will require a higher level of reasoning and analysis.

ii) **Comprehension:** Identify key concepts and/or facts in a passage. This will require you to infer, summarise and translate from the information presented.

iii) **Application:** Use the information presented in the passage to solve problems. This involves applying knowledge to new or existing problems presented in the stimulus/questions.

iv) **Analysis:** These types of questions require a holistic view of the stimulus and questions; they ask the candidate to organise ideas based on patterns and trends.

v) **Synthesis:** Use current information to create new ideas. Synthesis-style questions build further upon the inferences made in more basic comprehension questions, and often come after compre-hension questions within a unit. These questions ask candidates to make greater, more difficult inferences.

vi) **Evaluation:** These are the most cognitively challenging questions and require candi-dates to evaluate, judge and consider ideas or facts at a much higher and nuanced resolution. Often, many of the answer options will appear correct thus higher logic must be used to develop the answer in a process of elimination. Look out for words such as 'least', 'closest', 'most' as they tend to be used in this style of question.

3.4 Online Help

As most of you will come to learn, this textbook has ample practice material with worked solutions to develop and hone your Humanities and Social Sciences skills. For those of you who need more, there are other options. You can get Humanities and Social Sciences help online including over 20 mini-tests through GAMSAT University or the Platinum Package at GAMSAT-prep.com.

To access our latest suggestions for all GAMSAT sections including Humanities and Social Sciences, go to GAMSAT-prep.com and click FREE GAMSAT in the top menu.

High-level Importance

3.5 Types of Questions

Before we address the particular types of questions that you may be asked, it is useful to understand the nature of GAMSAT questions in general, and GAMSAT Humanities and Social Sciences questions in particular. Bloom's Taxonomy is an educational tool used to categorise questions that may be asked within an academic context. The levels of Bloom's model ascend according to the level of cognition required to answer particular questions. GAMSAT questions require candidates to exercise the levels leading towards the top of this model. Essentially, you will not be asked to simply recall or comprehend information you have read. Rather, the great majority of questions will require you to carry out complex cognitive tasks such as inferring, organising and evaluating.

The following is a list of typical question types you can expect to find as part of the Reasoning in Humanities and Social Sciences section of the GAMSAT. These questions may be asked within the context of different stimuli. As previously described, these stimuli include prose (extracts from literature, academic journals etc.), poetry and song lyrics, graphs and figures, cartoons and images, etc.

Main Idea Questions

These test your comprehension of the theme of the article. Questions may ask you for the main idea, central idea, purpose, a possible title for the passage, and so on. You may be asked to determine which statement best expresses the author's arguments or conclusions.

Please note that the styles of questions discussed in RHSS 3.3 correspond to the different levels of thinking skills in Bloom's Taxonomy, namely:

- Knowledge
- Comprehension
- Application
- Analysis
- Synthesis
- Evaluation

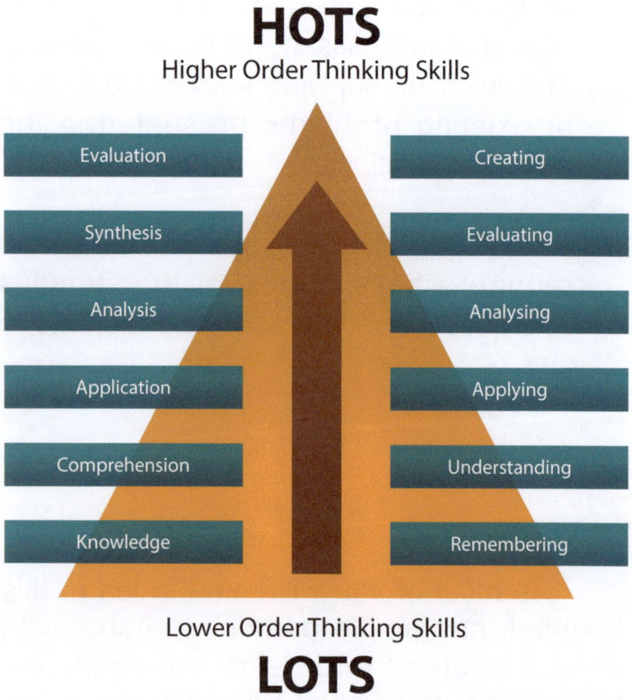

Figure 2: Bloom's original taxonomy on the left and revised taxonomy on the right (Anderson, Krathwohl 2002; Adapted from Tangient LLC 2014).

Inference Questions

These require you to understand the logic of the author's argument and then to decide what can be reasonably inferred from the article and what cannot be reasonably inferred. Occasionally, you will be asked to link like arguments/statements together into groups.

Analysis of Evidence Questions

These ask you to identify the evidence the author uses to support his/her argument. You may be required to analyse relationships between given and implied information. You may be asked not only to understand the way the author uses different pieces of information but also to evaluate whether the author has built sound arguments.

Implication Questions

You may be asked to make judgments about what would follow if the author is correct in his/her argument or what a particular discovery might lead to. You may be given new information and then asked how this affects the author's original argument.

Tone Questions

You may be asked to judge the attitude of the author towards the subject. The ability to understand tone also extends to comprehension of humour in its various guises including satire, lampoon, irony, hyperbole and parody among others (RHSS 3.5.5).

Hybrid Questions

Often more than one question type is used in the same instance. An "implication" question can be answered through the "tone" or "evidence" which is presented within the material. In addition, an assessment of material such as a "main idea" often includes "an analysis of evidence". There may be a number of "hybrid" type questions, which include one or more of all the question types discussed. In logically deducing and ruling out answers, two central ideas are very helpful: the most "encompassing" of the answers, and which of the answers has the most "explanatory power" in relation to the others. This will become more clear as we do some exercises.

3.5.1 Main Idea Questions

According to Bloom's Taxonomy, main idea questions ask candidates to utilise the intermediate skill of analysis which involves recognising and organising ideas into a hierarchy. These are therefore not the most difficult questions you will face in GAMSAT Humanities and Social Sciences, yet they are very important as they are quite prevalent.

We will do some exercises to ensure that you can successfully deal with these question types. Please take a piece of paper (i.e. Post-it note) to cover the answers while you are responding to the questions. The worked solutions and/or answers are upside down when appropriate. To find the main idea, ask the following three questions.

1. What is this passage about (the topic)?
2. What is the most important thing the author says about the topic (the main idea)?
3. Do all of the other ideas in the passage support this main idea?

Read the following passage and find the main idea.

For most immigrants, the journey to America was long and often full of hardships and suffering. The immigrants often walked the entire distance from their villages to the nearest seaport. There the ships might be delayed and precious time and money lost. Sometimes ticket agents or ship captains fleeced the immigrants of all they owned.

The most important idea in this paragraph is:

A. immigrants had to walk long distances to get to seaports.
B. ship schedules were very irregular.
C. ship captains often stole all the possessions of immigrants.
D. the journey of immigrants to America was very difficult and often painful.

1. *What is this passage about?*

____

____

2. *What is the most important thing the author says about the topic (the main idea)?*

____

____

3. *Do all of the other ideas in the passage support this main idea?*

____

____

1. This paragraph is about the immigrants' journey to America. This is the topic of the paragraph.
2. The author says that the immigrants' journey "was long and often full of hardships and suffering". This is the main idea of the paragraph.
3. To be absolutely sure that this is the main idea, ask yourself: Do all of the other ideas in the passage support this main idea? There are other ideas in the paragraph, but each one is an example of some kind of hardship suffered by the immigrants. Thus, the correct choice is D.

The Main Idea at the Beginning of a Passage

Did you notice that the main idea was contained in the first sentence? Often the main idea is in the first sentence. The main idea may also be contained in the title of a passage.

Read the following passage and find the main idea.

Working conditions in the factories were frequently unpleasant and dangerous. A workday of 14 or 16 hours was not uncommon. The work was uncertain. When the factory completed its orders, the men were laid off. Often the pay was inadequate to feed a man's family. This meant that often an entire family had to work in factories in order to survive.

This paragraph is most concerned with:

A. unfavourable and difficult working conditions in factories.

B. the passage of child-labour laws.

C. the lack of job security in early factories.

D. the low pay scale of early factories.

1. *What is this passage about?*

____

____

2. *What is the most important thing the author says about the topic (the main idea)?*

____

____

3. *Do all of the other ideas in the passage support this main idea?*

____

____

1. The topic of the passage is working conditions in the factories.
2. Working conditions in the factories were frequently dangerous and unpleasant.
3. All of the other sentences give examples of dangerous or unpleasant working conditions.

The correct choice is A.

Notice that all answer choices have an element of truth. However, the most encompassing, and therefore relevant, answer is A. Answer choices B, C and D are all specific examples of conditions included in A. In GAMSAT Humanities and Social Sciences, you may often be able to narrow your answer choices to two options. In these cases, always ensure you choose the most encompassing answer.

The Main Idea in the Middle of a Passage

Sometimes the main idea is stated somewhere in the middle of a paragraph. That is why the three questions about the main idea are so helpful.

What is this passage about? → *will help you focus on the main idea.*

What is the most important thing the author says about the topic? → *will point out the main idea.*

Do all of the other ideas in the passage support this main idea? → *will help you to be sure you have chosen the most important idea rather than one of the less important ideas.*

If you can answer these three questions, you will find the main idea no matter where it is placed in the paragraph.

Read the following passage carefully and ask yourself the three key questions. Then answer the question following the passage.

Many who had left the Catholic Church during the Protestant upheaval eventually returned to their original faith. However, the religious struggle of the sixteenth century destroyed the unity of Western Christendom. No longer was there one Church, nor one people, or one empire.

High-level Importance

The main point the author makes in this paragraph is that:

A. the Protestant Reformation destroyed the Catholic Church.

B. the Protestant Reformation did not affect the Catholic Church.

C. some Protestants rejoined the Catholic Church.

D. Western Christendom was never again unified after the Protestant Reformation.

1. *What is this passage about?*

____

____

2. *What is the most important thing the author says about the topic (the main idea)?*

____

____

3. *Do all of the other ideas in the passage support this main idea?*

____

____

The topic is the Protestant upheaval. The most important thing the author says about the Protestant upheaval is that it destroyed the unity of Western Christendom. The first sentence gives an example of unity. The second sentence points out that this example of unity was of minor importance compared to the disunity. The third sentence expands this idea of disunity and tells how extensive the disunity was. The main idea is contained in the second sentence. All of the other ideas support that sentence. Thus, the correct choice is D.

Answer choice A is close, however, it fails to address the specific notion of unity. Answer choice C is true, however, it is not the main idea. Answer choice B is simply incorrect.

The Main Idea in Several Sentences

The main idea is not always contained in a single sentence. Sometimes it takes more than one sentence to express a complex idea. Then you must piece together ideas from two or more sentences to find the main idea. The three questions are particularly helpful with paragraphs like this one:

Locke, of course, was no lone voice. The climate was right for him. He was a member of the Royal Society, and was thus intimately concerned with the work of the great seventeenth-century scientists. He argued that property, the possession of land and the making of money was a rational consequence of human freedom. This promise linked him to other great developments of the period: the formation of the powerful banks, the agricultural revolution, the new science, and the Industrial Revolution.

The main idea of this paragraph is:

A. John Locke believed that property was a product of human freedom.

B. John Locke was linked to the agricultural and industrial revolutions as well as to the new science and the formation of banks.

C. Property is the possession of land and the making of money.

D. John Locke's views on property linked him to all the other great developments of the seventeenth century.

1. *What is this passage about?*

____

____

2. *What is the most important thing the author says about the topic (the main idea)?*

____

____

3. *Do all of the other ideas in the passage support this main idea?*

____

____

You probably took a little more time to piece together the main idea. Notice that all of the choices are true statements. All of them are found in the passage. But now you are asked to judge which is the most important. The statement that includes all the main points of the passage should be the correct answer.

1. The topic is John Locke. More precisely, the passage is about how John Locke was linked to the great events of the seventeenth century.

2. What is the most important thing the author says about John Locke and the events of his time? Locke's idea that property was a natural result of human freedom linked him to the great developments of his period.

3. The first sentence says that Locke was not "a lone voice" which implies that his ideas were shared by many important people during his time. The second sentence complements this idea by saying that the "climate was right for him". These sentences support the idea that Locke was linked to the developments of his period. The third sentence states explicitly that Locke was "intimately concerned with the work of seventeenth-century scientists". The fourth sentence presents Locke's specific view on property (part of the main idea). The last sentence links Locke with the great developments of his period (part of the main idea) and it lists those developments. All of the sentences in the paragraph support the overarching idea that Locke's view on property linked him to several developments of his time. Answer choices A, B, and C support the main idea, but they do not state it completely. Choice D provides the most encompassing statement and is therefore correct.

The Main Idea in Several Paragraphs

So far, you have learned to find the main idea of paragraphs. To find the main idea of passages consisting of several paragraphs, first find the main idea of each paragraph. In the passage below, the main idea of each paragraph has been underlined.

Americans have long believed that George Washington died of injuries he received from a fall from a horse. <u>We now know that his doctors killed him.</u> Oh, it was no political assassination. They killed him by being what they were; physicians practicing good eighteenth-century medicine (which prescribed bleeding for every disease and injury). Washington was bled of two quarts of blood in two days.

It is commonly thought that the practice of blood-letting died with the eighteenth century, but even today leeches are sold in every major city in the United States. <u>These blood-sucking little worms are still used by ignorant people to draw off "bad blood,"</u> the old-world treatment for every disease of body and spirit.

The cities of America are infested with an even worse kind of bloodsucker than the leech. Like the leech, he is not a cure-all, but a cure-nothing. Like the leech, he transmits diseases more dangerous than those he is supposed to cure. And like his brother, the primordial worm, he kills more often than he cures. His name is "pusher". <u>His treatment is not blood-letting, but addiction.</u>

The purpose of the passage is to:

A. explain how George Washington died.
B. describe the eighteenth-century practice of using leeches to treat diseases.
C. denounce the practice of blood-letting.
D. make a comparison between leeches and drug pushers.

Re-read only the underlined portions of the passage. These sentences can be used to form a summary of the passage:

George Washington died of bleeding. Leeches are still used by ignorant people for treating diseases.

The cities of America are infested with an even worse kind of bloodsucker than the leech. His name is "pusher".

Now ask yourself the same questions you used to find the main idea of a single paragraph.

1. *What is this passage about?*

____

____

2. *What is the most important thing the author says about the topic (the main idea)?*

____

____

3. *Do all of the other ideas in the passage support this main idea?*

____

____

In addition to asking the three questions, you could also ask whether each of the answer choices is too narrow or too broad. For example, in the previous question choices A, B, and C are all too narrow to be the main idea.

1. The topic is leeches, blood-letting, and drug pushers.
2. Drug pushers are worse than leeches and do more harm than blood-letting.
3. The first paragraph explains that leeches were used in the eighteenth century and could kill people. The second paragraph explains that ignorant people still use leeches. The third paragraph compares leeches and drug pushers and stresses that drugs are the more harmful. The answer is D.

3.5.2 Inference Questions

Some questions ask you to make inferences. An inference is a conclusion not directly stated in the text but implied by it.

Referring back to Bloom's Taxonomy, inferences is a high-level cognitive skill considered to be a component of Synthesis in the original taxonomy, and a component of Creating in the revised taxonomy. Inferring may also extend to extrapolating upon a particular idea, or sentiment. These types of questions can be complex.

Read the following passage. The topic is not directly stated, but you can infer what the paragraph is about.

Dark clouds moved swiftly across the sky blotting out the sun. With no further warning, great cracks of thunder and flashes of lightning disturbed the morning's calm. Fortunately, the deckhands had already tied everything securely in place and closed all portholes and hatches or we would have lost our gear to the fury of wind and water.

1. This passage most likely describes:

- **A.** a storm during an African safari.
- **B.** a storm at sea.
- **C.** an Antarctic expedition.
- **D.** a flash flood.

2. Which of the following statements is false?

- **A.** The storm was unexpected.
- **B.** The storm came suddenly.
- **C.** It was windy.
- **D.** It was cloudy.

The words dark clouds, thunder, lightning, wind, and water all suggest a storm. The words deckhands and portholes suggest a ship at sea. The answer to question 1 is B.

Nowhere in the paragraph are the words "sudden storm at sea" but, obviously, that is what the paragraph is about. Several other words give you the feeling of the suddenness of the storm. On the other hand, are you justified in concluding that the storm was unexpected? You know that things that happen suddenly are often unexpected. Was that the case with this storm? The last sentence tells you that the deckhands had already tied everything down and closed all portholes and hatches. That sentence indicates the storm, while sudden, was expected. The answer to question 2 is A.

Note that Answer A is a false statement and that's why it is the correct answer. Students often make mistakes with double negative questions (i.e. the question is asking for something false and the answer has "unexpected"). Process of elimination (3.2.4) and annotating your scratch paper (i.e. noting down wrong options or likely correct answers, whichever suits the case) will reduce the chance that you will make a mental error.

Read the following paragraph. You will be asked to examine the cause-effect relationships implied by it later.

Effect of Position on Valsalva Maneuver: Supine vs. 20-Degree Position

Blood pressure (BP) changes in response to the Valsalva manoeuvre (VM), which reflects the integrity of the baroreflex that regulates BP. Performing this manoeuvre in the standard supine position often prevents adequate venous preload reduction, resulting in a rise rather than a fall in BP, the "flat top" Valsalva response. We determined whether performing the Valsalva Maneuver (VM) at a 20-degree angle of head up tilt improves preload reduction, thereby reducing the frequency of flat top responses, improving reflex vasoconstriction, and increasing the Valsalva ratio (VR). 130 patients were evaluated in a prospective study. Each patient performed the VM in both supine and 20-degree positions.

Flat top responses were present in 18% of subjects when supine. Twenty-degree position reduced the flat top response by 87%. The components of the response that are dependent on preload reduction also showed significant improvement with the 20-degree position.

A 20-degree angle of tilt is sufficient to reduce venous preload, decreasing flat top response rate and improving the VR and the morphology of the VM. We recommend this modification for laboratory evaluation of the VM, whenever a "flat-top" response is seen.

(PMC2729588; 2009)

3. The "flat top" response is triggered by:

A. a high preload reduction.
B. a rise in blood pressure.
C. supine performance of the VM.
D. performance of the VM with 20-degree head tilt.

In this case, there are many concepts that are likely to be foreign to the candidate. Rest assured, you do not require prior knowledge of such concepts to answer such questions. In this case, the correct answer is C. A is incorrect because it is actually a low preload reduction that causes the flat top response. B is incorrect as a rise in blood pressure is in fact what constitutes the flat top response. Finally, D is incorrect as the 20-degree head tilt is the method that the study shows reduces the prevalence of the "flat top" response.

Read the following paragraph. The question following it is concerned with the relationships between the main idea and supporting details.

Do we live in a revolutionary age? Our television and newspapers seem to tell us that we do. The late twentieth century has seen the governments of China and Cuba, among others, overthrown. The campuses of our universities erupted into violence; above the confusion of voices could be heard slogans of social revolution. We are constantly reminded that we live in a time of scientific and technological revolution. Members of militant racial groups cry for the necessity and inevitability of violent revolution. Even a new laundry detergent is described as "revolutionary!" Many causes, many voices, all use the same word.

4. Revolutionary ages are generally marked by:

A. violence, slogans, science.
B. violence, television coverage, governments overthrown.
C. peace, science, technology.
D. violence, confusion, governments overthrown.

Notice that the author does not answer his own question in the first sentence (the main idea). All of the other sentences give illustrations or examples of "revolution". The question asks you to make a generalisation about the nature of revolution from these examples. Choices A and B include examples from a particular revolution (if one does exist). They are not true generalisations. Choice C is patently contrary to the ideas of the passage. Choice D is correct.

3.5.3 Analysis of Evidence Questions

Some questions ask you to check back in the text to see if the passage confirms or refutes a particular detail. This is the easiest kind of question to answer. In fact, the answer may be so obvious, you may be tempted to feel that some kind of trick is involved. Relax! If you can find the answer in the passage, you are almost certainly right.

While it will not be as simple as just comprehending a particular fact, often only basic insight is required. The trick here may be to watch for double negatives, or the understanding of particular or sophisticated vocabulary.

Do not worry if you learn new words during your GAMSAT preparation. That's normal! The majority of students will learn many new words and expressions while studying for RHSS. If you don't, then you are probably not practising enough (or you have unusually advanced English skills). Be sure to take notes for your RHSS preparation, just as you would for Written Communication and Sciences. Study from your notes often.

Attempt the following questions relating to the poem Beat! Beat! Drums! by Walt Whitman.

Beat! Beat! Drums! by Walt Whitman

Beat! beat! drums!—Blow! bugles! blow!
Through the windows—through the doors—burst like a force of armed men,
Into the solemn church, and scatter the congregation;
Into the school where the scholar is studying;
Leave not the bridegroom quiet—no happiness must he have now with his bride;
Nor the peaceful farmer any peace plowing his field or gathering his grain;
So fierce you whirr and pound, you drums—so shrill you bugles blow.

Beat! beat! drums! Blow! bugles! blow!
Over the traffic of cities—over the rumble of wheels in the streets;
Are beds prepared for sleepers at night in the houses? No sleepers must sleep in those beds;
No bargainers' bargains by day—no brokers or speculators. Would they continue?
Would the talkers be talking? would the singer attempt to sing?
Would the lawyer rise in the court to state his case before the judge?
Then rattle quicker, heavier drums—and bugles wilder blow.

Beat! beat! drums! Blow! bugles! blow!
Make no parley—stop for no expostulation;
Mind not the timid—mind not the weeper or prayer;
Mind not the old man beseeching the young man;
Let not the child's voice be heard, nor the mother's entreaties. Recruit! recruit!
Make the very trestles shake under the dead, where they lie in their shrouds awaiting the hearses.
So strong you thump, O terrible drums—so loud you bugles blow.

5. The poem relates an instance of which of the following?
- **A.** Conscription for war
- **B.** Propaganda dictated by authority
- **C.** Commercial infiltration of daily life
- **D.** Spawning of a social revolution

6. In the context of the poem, which of the following is closest in meaning to 'expostulation'?
- **A.** Confirmation
- **B.** Remonstration
- **C.** Exclamation
- **D.** Negotiation

7. The author uses many persons to emphasise his point. Which of these combinations is not used by the author?
- **A.** Clergy, fathers and children
- **B.** Mothers, children and those who perished
- **C.** Businessmen, farmers and physicians
- **D.** Brides, mothers and the judiciary

Question 5 clearly relates to war, thus the answer is A. The words bugle (the small trumpet often used for military signals), recruit and references to the dead on trestles (eventually, hearses) all support this notion. Note that the instruments are "loud" and "terrible" like war itself. Answer choices B, C and D could be assumed, but are not supported by evidence in the passage.

Question 6 asks you to define the term expostulation in context. Given the careless, relentless and advancing nature of the piece, B is the correct answer. Expostulation, or remonstration in this context, refers to disagreeing or arguing about something. Answer choices A and D are close, but fail to encompass the sentiment of the use of the word. Answer choice C can be ruled out easily as incorrect.

Question 7 is a basic comprehension question. All combinations within answer choices A, B and D are used by Whitman in the poem. Answer choice C is the correct answer as the author makes no reference to physicians while stressing the undiscriminating recruitment drive for war.

3.5.4 Implication Questions

Sometimes you will have to apply one of the ideas in a passage to another situation. Sometimes this type of question takes a broad generalisation from the passage and asks you to apply it to a specific situation. In the context of Bloom's Taxonomy, this involves the higher cognitive skill of synthesis. Attempt the passage below.

In December 1946, full-scale war broke out between French soldiers and Viet Minh forces. The people tended to support the Viet Minh. Communist countries aided the rebels, especially after 1949 communist regime came to power in China. The United States became involved in the struggle in 1950, when the United States declared support of Vietnamese independence, under Bao Dai.

Finally, in 1954, at the battle of Dien Bien Phu, the French suffered a shattering defeat and decided to withdraw. The 1954 Geneva Conference, which arranged for a ceasefire, provisionally divided Vietnam into northern and southern sectors at the 17th parallel. The unification of Vietnam was to be achieved by general elections to be held in July 1956 in both sectors under international supervision. In the north, the Democratic Republic of Vietnam was led by its president, Ho Chi Minh, and was dominated by the Communist Party.

In the south, Ngo Dinh Diem took over the government when Bao Dai left the country in 1954. As the result of a referendum held in 1955, a republic was established in South Vietnam, with Diem as President.

High-level Importance

8. A good title for this passage would be (main idea question):

- **A.** "The United States and Vietnam"
- **B.** "The Geneva Conference"
- **C.** "The Vietnamese Fight for Independence"
- **D.** "The Career of Bao Dai"

9. In the second paragraph, the word "provisionally" means (implication question):

- **A.** temporarily.
- **B.** permanently.
- **C.** with a large, outfitted army.
- **D.** helplessly.

10. Bao Dai was in 1950 (implication question):

- **A.** a possible Vietnamese independence leader.
- **B.** the leader of the French.
- **C.** the brother of Dien Bien Phu.
- **D.** the President of South Vietnam.

11. The tone of this passage is (tone question):

- **A.** objective.
- **B.** partial to the French.
- **C.** partial to the North Vietnamese.
- **D.** cynical.

12 . From the passage, we might assume that in 1946, the Viet Minh were (implication question):

- **A.** South Vietnamese.
- **B.** Vietnamese rebels.
- **C.** North Vietnamese.
- **D.** French-supporting Vietnamese.

8. C
9. A
10. A
11. A
12. B

3.5.5 Tone Questions

An author may express his feelings or attitudes toward a subject. This expression of emotion imparts a tone to the writing. To determine the tone of a passage, think of the emotions or attitudes that are expressed throughout the passage. Below are some terms that can be used on the exam to describe tone.

Term	Meaning
Admiring	respectful, approving
Belittling	making small, depreciating

Term	Meaning
Cynical	unbelieving, sneering
Denigrating	blackening, defamatory
Didactic	instructive, authoritarian
Ebullient	exuberant, praising
Hyperbolic	overstated, exaggerating
Ironic	incongruous, contrasting
Lampooning	satirical, making fun of
Laudatory	praising

Term	Meaning
Mendacious	untruthful, lying
Objective	factual
Optimistic	hopeful
Praising	commending, laudatory
Reverential	exalted, regarding as sacred
Ridiculing	deriding, mocking, scornful
Saddened	sorrowful, mournful
Sanguine	confident, hopeful
Sarcastic	bitter, ironic
Sardonic	mocking, bitter, cynical
Satiric	ridiculing, mocking
Tragic	sad

A tragic tone reflects misfortune and unfulfilled hopes. A satiric tone mocks and ridicules its subject. An author may use an ironic tone to develop a contrast between **(1)** what is said and what is meant, **(2)** what actually happens and what appears to be happening, or **(3)** what happens and what was expected to happen. These are just a few of the emotions or attitudes that influence the tone.

Words themselves, statements and the general sentiment of the author all contribute to tone. Thus when attempting any GAMSAT Humanities and Social Sciences question, ensure you maintain awareness of the tone of the author. Even if there are no questions directly asking about tone, tone is likely to have a bearing upon how you approach other questions, especially when the stimulus is poetry, literature, or journalistic.

Attempt the questions below.

A certain rugby team won a regional championship for the first time in many years. Different people reacted differently.

13. "Wow! I can't believe it! This is the best thing that could have happened in this city!"
The tone of this remark is:
- **A.** serious.
- **B.** excited.
- **C.** sarcastic.
- **D.** amazed.

14. "Ah! This is like it was when I was a boy. It makes my chest swell with pride again and brings tears to my eyes."
The tone of this remark is:
- **A.** sentimental.
- **B.** excited.
- **C.** sarcastic.
- **D.** amazed.

15. "The team's manager and coach have had a lot of influence throughout the season. They deserve a lot of credit for this victory."
The tone of this remark is:
- **A.** serious.
- **B.** excited.
- **C.** sarcastic.
- **D.** amazed.

High-level Importance

16. "What!? They won!? And they started off so poorly this season. I just can't believe it!"
The tone of this remark is:
- **A.** serious.
- **B.** excited.
- **C.** sarcastic.
- **D.** amazed.

17. "It couldn't have been skill since they don't have that. It couldn't have been bribery, since they don't have any money. The other team must all have been sick. It's the only way they could have won."
The tone of this remark is:
- **A.** serious.
- **B.** excited.
- **C.** sarcastic.
- **D.** amazed.

13. B
14. A
15. A
16. D
17. C

3.6 Warm-up Exercises

These short, relatively easy passages will help consolidate the principles and techniques explained in RHSS 3.5.

Passage 12

As the mid-century approached, the women of America were far from being acclimated to their assigned dependent role. In fact, leaders of the growing suffrage movement were seeking equality under the law. Incredible as it seems now, in early nineteenth-century America a wife, like a black slave, could not lawfully retain title to property after marriage. She could not vote, and she could legally be beaten by her master.

18. One of the goals of the suffrage movement was:
- **A.** dependence on a master.
- **B.** equality with men.
- **C.** recognition of divorce.
- **D.** abolition of slavery.

19. Which sentence describes American women of the early 19th century?
- **A.** They were against marriage.
- **B.** They were satisfied with their role in society.
- **C.** They were victims of a male-dominated society.
- **D.** They had many slaves to do their work.

18. B
19. C

Passage 13

No dwelling in all the world stirs the imagination like the tipi of the Plains Indian. It is without doubt one of the most picturesque of all shelters and one of the most practical movable dwellings ever invented. Comfortable, roomy, and well ventilated, it was ideal for the roving life these people led in following the buffalo herds up and down the country. It also proved to be just as ideal in a more permanent camp during the long winters on the prairies.

20. What is a tlpi?
- **A.** A buffalo
- **B.** An Indian
- **C.** A prairie
- **D.** A residence

21. What kind of life did the Plains Indians lead?
- **A.** They wandered with the buffaloes.
- **B.** They led comfortable and ideal lives.
- **C.** They spent their lives in one place.
- **D.** They lived in large, airy caves.

20. D
21. A

Passage 14

A dozen years ago, Thornton Wilder and I made the happy discovery that we were both invited to a White House dinner for the French Minister of Culture, Andre Malraux. We decided at once to go together. He was to pick up my wife and me at our hotel, and specified that I should have a double old-fashioned ready for him. Thornton did justice to the drink. He also delighted my wife. She was nervous about the dress she was wearing, and he told her it reminded him of the black swan of Tasmania and was so graceful that it danced almost by itself. He illustrated in long, slow undulations, his arms waving. My wife was ham all evening.

22. Who is the narrator of the passage?
- **A.** Andre Malraux
- **B.** Thornton Wilder
- **C.** The passage does not say.
- **D.** Tasmania

23. What does "happy" mean in the expression "happy discovery"?
- **A.** Fortunate
- **B.** Contented
- **C.** Optimistic
- **D.** Clever

24. What delighted the narrator's wife?
- **A.** The invitation to the White House
- **B.** Wilder's compliment
- **C.** A double old-fashioned
- **D.** Attending the dinner with Wilder

22. C
23. A
24. B

Passage 15

Nobody knows with certainty how big a proportion of the world's population is suffering from the basic problem of chronic undernourishment. But the commonly quoted

United Nations estimate of 460 million sufferers is, if anything, on the low side. This represents 15 percent of the global population. Many more suffer from other deficiencies, making global totals even more difficult to calculate.

25. The paragraph indicates that:
- **A.** malnutrition is the number one problem in modern society.
- **B.** relatively few people suffer from malnutrition.
- **C.** the United Nations is supplying food to those suffering from malnutrition.
- **D.** it is not easy to count the number of people in the world who are undernourished.

25. D

Passage 16

Another way to fight insomnia is to exercise every day. Muscular relaxation is an important part of sleep. Daily exercise leaves your muscles pleasantly relaxed and ready for sleep.

26. What is insomnia?
- **A.** Muscular relaxation
- **B.** Inability to sleep
- **C.** Exercise
- **D.** Sleep

27. According to the passage, daily exercise:
- **A.** helps a person fall asleep more readily.
- **B.** is harmful to the muscles.
- **C.** prepares a person for fighting.
- **D.** is unnecessary.

26. B
27. A

Passage 17

The decade was erected upon the smouldering wreckage of the '60s. Now and then, someone's shovel blade would strike an unexploded bomb; mostly the air in the '70s was thick with a sense of aftermath, of public passions spent and consciences bewildered. The American gaze turned inward. It distracted itself with diversions trivial or squalid. The U.S. lost a President and a war, and not only endured those unique humiliations with grace, but showed enough resilience to bring a Roman-candle burst of spirit to its Bicentennial celebration.

28. What image is used to describe the '70s?
- **A.** A celebration
- **B.** A race
- **C.** A postwar period
- **D.** A long movie full of passion

29. What is the author's attitude regarding the events of the '70s?
- **A.** He is pessimistic.
- **B.** He is bewildered.
- **C.** He is optimistic.
- **D.** He is afraid.

28. C
29. C

Passage 18

One bright spot in the U.S. economy in 1979 was the surprising decline in gasoline use. Rising fuel costs are finally prodding Americans to cut back on consumption, and the need for this becomes more acute all the time.

30. How does the author view the decline in gas consumption?

A. He is indifferent.
B. He thinks it is a good sign.
C. He doesn't see the need for it.
D. He is unhappy about it.

31. Why are Americans using less gasoline?

A. The economy is good.
B. They do not need as much.
C. They want to spend more time at home.
D. Gasoline is becoming very expensive.

30. B
31. D

Passage 19

During the early part of the colonial period, living conditions were hard, and people had little leisure time for reading or studying. Books imported from abroad were expensive and were bought mainly by ministers, lawyers, and wealthy merchants. The only books to be found in most homes were the Bible and an almanac, a book giving general information about such subjects as astronomy, the weather, and farming.

32. The early colonists did not do much reading because:

A. they did not know how to read.
B. the Bible told them that reading was sinful.
C. they did not have time.
D. they were not interested in reading.

33. Books were bought primarily by:

A. the nobility.
B. professional and wealthy people.
C. the lower class.
D. sellers of almanacs.

32. C
33. B

Passage 20

Never before in history have people been so aware of what is going on in the world. Television, newspapers, radio keep us continually informed and stimulate our interest. The sociologist's interest in the world around him is intense, for society is his field of study. As an analyst, he must be well acquainted with a broad range of happenings and must understand basic social processes. He wants to know what makes the social world what it is, how it is organised, why it changes in the way that it does. Such knowledge is valuable not only for those who make great decisions, but also for you, since this is the world in which you live and make your way.

34. The passage chiefly concerns:
- **A.** the work of a sociologist.
- **B.** the news media.
- **C.** modern society.
- **D.** decision-makers.

35. It can be inferred that a good sociologist must be:
- **A.** persistent.
- **B.** sensitive.
- **C.** objective.
- **D.** curious.

36. According to the passage, modern society is more aware of world events than were previous societies because:
- **A.** the news media keep us better informed.
- **B.** travel is easier and faster.
- **C.** there are more analysts.
- **D.** today's population is more sociable.

34. A
35. D
36. A

Passage 21

Whatever answer the future holds, this much I believe we must accept: there can be no putting the genie back into the bottle. To try to bury or to suppress new knowledge because we do not know how to prevent its use for destructive or evil purposes is a pathetically futile gesture. It is, indeed, a symbolic return to the methods of the Middle Ages. It seeks to deny the innermost urge of the mind of men; the desire for knowledge.

37. The author believes that:
- **A.** new ideas should not be encouraged.
- **B.** we should return to the methods of the Middle Ages.
- **C.** new knowledge is always used for evil purposes.
- **D.** to suppress knowledge is a useless act.

38. What is the meaning of "no putting the genie back into the bottle"?
- **A.** Once new discoveries have been made, it is impossible to deny their existence and to control the consequences which might result from them.
- **B.** We cannot be sure that knowledge will be used for humanitarian purposes.
- **C.** The desire for knowledge was not strong during the Middle Ages.
- **D.** We cannot answer tomorrow's questions today.

39. According to the author, man's most basic desire is:
- **A.** to know the future.
- **B.** to prevent destruction and evil.
- **C.** to become less ignorant.
- **D.** to avoid useless activity.

40. The passage was written:

- **A.** to convince us that the Middle Ages contributed little to modern society.
- **B.** to inspire us to meet challenges wisely.
- **C.** to persuade us to mistrust new ideas.
- **D.** to show us what we can expect in the future.

37. D
38. A
39. C
40. B This answer remains after eliminating the others.

Passage 22

It is important to distinguish among communication, language, and speech. These terms may, of course, be used synonymously, but strictly speaking, communication refers to the transmission or reception of a message, while language, which is usually used interchangeably with speech, is here taken to mean the speech of a population viewed as an objective entity, whether reduced to writing or in any other form.

41. According to the author, which word could be best used to replace "speech"?

- **A.** Communication
- **B.** Transmission
- **C.** Language
- **D.** Reception

42. The author understands "language" to mean:

- **A.** the totality of the way a given people expresses itself.
- **B.** the giving or receiving of a message.
- **C.** the exchange of words between two people.
- **D.** the written works of a population.

41. C
42. A

Passage 23

The long, momentous day of John Glenn began at 2:20 a.m. when he was awakened in his simple quarters at Cape Canaveral's hangars by the astronauts' physician, Dr. William K. Douglas. Glenn had slept a little over seven hours. He shaved, showered, and breakfasted. Outside, the moon was obscured by fleecy clouds; the weather, responsible for four of the nine previous postponements, looked rather ominous.

43. At approximately what time did Glenn go to sleep?

- **A.** 5 p.m.
- **B.** 7 p.m.
- **C.** 9 a.m.
- **D.** 7 a.m.

44. Which statement about the weather is true?

- **A.** It was perfect for the occasion.
- **B.** It was cloudy and rainy.
- **C.** It had caused delays in the past.
- **D.** The passage does not say.

High-level Importance

45. Who is John Glenn?

A. A doctor
B. A weatherman
C. A spaceman
D. A sailor

43. B
44. C
45. C

Passage 24

Freud wrote several important essays on literature, which he used to explore the psyche of authors and characters, to explain narrative mysteries, and to develop new concepts in psychoanalysis (for instance, *Delusion and Dream in Jensen's Gradiva* and his influential readings of the Oedipus myth and Shakespeare's *Hamlet in The Interpretation of Dreams*). The criticism has been made, however, that in his and his early followers' studies "what calls for elucidation are not the artistic and literary works themselves, but rather the psychopathology and biography of the artist, writer or fictional characters." Thus many psychoanalysts among Freud's earliest adherents did not resist the temptation to psychoanalyse poets and painters sometimes to Freud's chagrin. Later analysts would conclude that "clearly one cannot psychoanalyse a writer from his text; one can only appropriate him."

46. What would be the best title for this passage?

A. Freudian Analysis of Literary Works
B. The Interdisciplinary Work of Freud on Classical Literature
C. Criticisms on the Psychoanalysis of Literature
D. Pitfalls of Psychoanalysis in Art and Literature

47. With which statement would the author of the passage agree?

A. Freud's work has been influential both in psychology and literature.
B. One cannot always conclude about a writer's psyche based on his literary work alone.
C. Many psychoanalysts were wrong in their findings of art and literature.
D. Psychology and Literature can never go hand in hand.

48. Which of the following would Freud NOT be interested in analysing?

A. painters
B. writers
C. psychological novels
D. fictional characters

46. C
47. B
48. C

SPOILER ALERT

Gold Standard has cross-referenced the content in this chapter to examples from ACER's official GAMSAT practice materials. It is for you to decide when you want to explore these questions since you may want to preserve some of ACER's materials for timed mock-exam practice.

Examples – Main Idea Questions Q3 of 1; Q2, Q13, Q15 of 2; Q2, Q5, Q8-10, Q17, Q26-29, Q30, Q47, Q53-55, Q75 of 3; Q15, Q24-25, Q31, 45, 72 of 4; Q7 and 8, Q10, Q17 and 18, Q28, Q44, Q66, Q68 of 5; Inference Questions Q7, Q8, Q21, Q27 of 1; Q18-21 of 2; Q22, Q33 and Q35, Q38 and 39, Q63 of 3; Q1-6, Q16-17, Q18-20, Q22-23 and Q26, 27, 29, Q38-39, Q46-54 of 4; Q15, Q34, Q48, Q50-54 of 5; Analysis of Evidence Questions Q24, 31 of 1; Q4, Q6 of 2; Q3, Q13, Q44 of 3; Q9-10, 37, 40, 58 of 4; Q11, Q23, Q30, Q35, Q45, Q59 of 5; Tone Questions Q10, Q14-Q18 of 1; Q22 and Q30 of 2; Q43, Q62 of 3; Q12, 16, 20, Q21, Q41 and 43, Q70 of 5; Implication Questions Q6, Q22, Q29 of 1; Q18-21 of 3; Q41 of 4; Q49, Q61, Q73 of 5; Hybrid Questions Q35 of 1; Q16 of 2; Q12, Q36 and 37, Q56-60 of 3; Q65 of 4; Q74-75 of 5. Note that "Q" is followed by the question number, and, for example, "of 1" refers to booklet number 1 which is referenced in the Spoiler Alert table at the end of section RHSS 3.2.4. The 15 full-length HEAPS GAMSAT practice tests (by Gold Standard) include exams that contain specific cross-references to this chapter within the worked solutions.

Chapter Checklist

- ☐ Access your online account to view answers, worked solutions and discussion boards.
- ☐ Complete a maximum of 1 page of notes using symbols/abbreviations to represent the content in the foregoing section. These are your Gold Notes.
- ☐ Consider your options based on your optimal way of learning:
  - ☐ Create your own, tangible study cards or try the free app: Anki.
  - ☐ Record your voice reading your Gold Notes onto your smartphone (MP3s) and listen during exercise, transportation, etc.
  - ☐ Consider reading at least 1 source material every day (e.g., poems of a single author, a synopsis of a novel, an article from a scientific journal that caught your interest, etc.). Note down the main idea or ideas of the piece on your scratch paper. Determine or surmise the author's sentiment or purpose for writing the material.
- ☐ Reassess your schedule for your full-length GAMSAT practice tests: ACER and/or HEAPS exams. Ensure that you have scheduled one full day to complete a practice test and 1-2 days for a thorough assessment of worked solutions while adding to your abbreviated Gold Notes.
- ☐ Reassess your progress in scheduling and/or evaluating stress reduction techniques such as regular exercise (sports), yoga, meditation and/or mindfulness exercises (*see* YouTube for suggestions).

3.7 Short Test and Analysis

The multiple-choice Humanities and Social Sciences of the GAMSAT, as described before, is organised into Units. Now that you have worked through all the warm-up exercises, you can proceed to test yourself with GAMSAT-style Units with appropriate stimulus material. We will work through the answers when you are finished.

There are 7 Units with 15 questions: choose the best answer for each question. Based on the timing introduced by ACER for the very first time in 2022, you have 24 minutes (*this amounts to an average of 1.6 minutes per question*). Please time yourself.

BEGIN ONLY WHEN TIMER IS READY.

Unit 1

Questions 1–2

Marked by a rise of technology, the global economy can be thought of as a complex international system, interlinked through the flow of goods, services, and information. Geographically, there are spatial changes, in labour and production, and the global economy is marked by a lifting of trade barriers and restrictions. Globalisation has to some extent levelled out the competitive labour between major industrial countries and emerging countries. While prior to globalisation, the United States dominated the global economy to a great extent, with the advent of information technologies, such as computers, the internet and the Web, the relocation of jobs from high-wage to low-wage countries, the emergence of economic blocs, such as NAFTA, and the nascent beginning of industrialisation in Southeast Asia, the U.S. is purportedly dwindled to roughly one quarter of the global economy's flow of goods, services and information.

1. The best metaphor in describing the global economy in the passage would be:

- **A.** medium.
- **B.** river.
- **C.** network.
- **D.** hypertext.

2. One can make the inference that the spatial changes in labour and production are not only due to the lifting of trade barriers and restrictions but also because of:
   A. the production of goods and services in the US only.
   B. the advent of information technologies, such as the internet.
   C. the rise of the minimum wage in the United States.
   D. the displacement of labour due to economic factors.

Unit 2

Question 3

Oxymorons are literary devices, which bring two contradictory terms together to establish a nuance of meaning, or use, for effect. The rhetorical term oxymoron, made up of two Greek words meaning "sharp" and "dull", is itself oxymoronic. "Cheerful pessimist", "wise fool", and "sad joy" are all examples of oxymorons. This device is used in literary classics but also in everyday speech. "The true beauty of oxymorons," says Richard Watson Todd, "is that, unless we sit back and really think, we happily accept them as normal English." Todd illustrates his point in the following passage:

> *It was an open secret that the company had used a paid volunteer to test the plastic glasses. Although they were made using liquid gas technology and were an original copy that looked almost exactly like a more expensive brand, the volunteer thought that they were pretty ugly and that it would be simply impossible for the general public to accept them. On hearing this feedback, the company board was clearly confused and there was a deafening silence. This was a minor crisis and the only choice was to drop the product line.*

(Much Ado About English. Nicholas Brealey Publishing, 2006)

3. Given the description about oxymorons, which of the following phrases could LEAST be considered an oxymoron?
   A. Unbiased opinion
   B. Devout atheist
   C. Tough predicament
   D. Idiot savant

Unit 3

Questions 4–5

Morning at the Window

They are rattling breakfast plates in basement kitchens,
And along the trampled edges of the street
I am aware of the damp souls of housemaids
Sprouting despondently at area gates.
The brown waves of fog toss up to me
Twisted faces from the bottom of the street,
And tear from a passer-by with muddy skirts
An aimless smile that hovers in the air
And vanishes along the level of the roofs.

T.S. Eliot

4. The images described by the speaker in the poem suggest:
- **A.** poverty and dejection among the lower class.
- **B.** hope despite misery among the lower class.
- **C.** a juxtaposition of the lower class and the upper class.
- **D.** a busy start of the day.

5. Which of the following observations about T.S. Eliot's style of poetry best characterises the quality of "Morning at the Window"?

"Morning at the Window" presents:
- **A.** an interpretation of a meditated experience.
- **B.** a quiet yet involved desperation of sentiments.
- **C.** images that describe the poet's sentiments toward a social condition.
- **D.** an aggregation of images that evoke an emotional response in the reader.

Unit 4

Questions 6–10

Cyberterrorism, simply defined, is a convergence of computers, the internet, and terrorism. A specialist in cyberterrorism, Dorothy Denning, defines cyberterrorism as, "unlawful attacks and threats of attack against computers, networks, and the information stored therein when done to intimidate or coerce a government or its people in furtherance of political or social objectives". Further, to qualify as cyberterrorism, an attack should result in violence against persons or property, or at least cause enough harm to generate fear.

To some extent, differentiation is made between cyber crimes, such as phishing and cyber sapping from cyberterrorism, but the line of demarcation becomes less accurate when major corporations are being hacked into.

The line between the two usually focusses on the "level of danger" or "threat" which is usually not an individual hacker but a "premeditated use of disruptive activities, or the threat thereof, against computers and/or networks, with the intention to cause harm or further social, ideological, religious, political or similar objectives, or to intimidate any person in furtherance of such objectives." This definition is a merger of cyber and definitions of terrorism by the United States Department of Defense. The line between cyber crime and cyberterrorism becomes quite arbitrary when considering that such a "cyber crime" as "identity theft" could be used by a terrorist to establish another identity or multiple identities. The use of bots, malware, spyware, viruses, and worms, provides another example in which one must distinguish whether the purported use on computer networks is by an alienated teenager or a terrorist.

Many countries (U.S., U.K., and India) will admit to "hacking" or internet intrusions from the same suspects: China and/or Russia, and admit that the internet must be thought of as a utility, in the same manner as water, power, and possibly vulnerable to cyber-attack. There have been other "intrusions" in the past few years. The U.S. Power grid was invaded by software (by China or Russia), Estonia, Chechnya and Kyrgyzstan have all come under cyber attack, an estranged employee dumped massive amounts of sewage in Australia through a rigged computer program, air control traffic in Alaska was hacked, causing a partial shutdown of the airport. These are notable examples that are quite real to those who would proclaim that cyberterrorism is a myth. "Hackers" theorise an attack on vulnerable businesses and corporations within the infrastructure of countries, instead of government "intrusions". One has to admit that the private sector and government sector are intertwined, interdependent, and possibly vulnerable to cyberterrorism.

6. According to the passage, the difference between "cyber crime" and "cyberterrorism" seems to be:
   - **A.** congruous.
   - **B.** tenuous.
   - **C.** categorical.
   - **D.** well-defined.

7. The author of the passage can be inferred to be:
   - **A.** strongly opposed to hacking and cyber crime.
   - **B.** indifferent towards the concept of cyberterrorism.
   - **C.** opinionated yet professional on the issue of cyberterrorism.
   - **D.** impartial towards the concept of cyberterrorism.

8. Which of the following can be inferred as the reason why the internet must be thought of as a public utility, much the same as water or power (lines 21-22)?
   - **A.** It is run by both public and private companies.
   - **B.** Governments and the internet are connected.
   - **C.** It could be a likely target for terrorism.
   - **D.** Most of the developed countries have access to the internet.

9. Which of the following arguments from the passage can be used to dispute the opinion that cyberterrorism is a myth?
   - **A.** Real wars can be fought through the use of the internet.
   - **B.** There is a difference between cyber crime and cyberterrorism.
   - **C.** Cyberterrorism can blow up buildings and kill people.
   - **D.** Cyberterrorism can cause public harm and fear.

10. What does the author mean by "infrastructure" in line 28?
   - **A.** The vulnerable aspects of digital networks
   - **B.** The digital networks of private enterprise
   - **C.** The digital networks of private and public enterprise
   - **D.** The digital networks of public enterprise

Unit 5

Question 11

A literary critic once remarked that the whole point of reading the works of Franz Kafka was to re-read. Indeed, Kafka presents an abstract world of images which almost seem to operate on their own volition.

The following are two very short stories by Franz Kafka.

The Wish to be a Red Indian

If one were only an Indian, instantly alert, and on a racing horse, leaning against the wind, kept on quivering jerkily over the quivering ground, until one shed one's spurs, for there needed no spurs, threw away the reins, for there needed no reins, and hardly saw that the land before one was smoothly shorn heath when horse's neck and head would be already gone.

The Trees

For we are like tree trunks in the snow. In appearance they lie sleekly and a little push should be enough to set them rolling. No, it can't be done, for they are firmly wedded to the ground. But see, even that is only appearance.

11. Which of the following terms would best describe the two stories, respectively?

A. Initiation – Naturalisation
B. Aspiration – Perception
C. Alienation – Transformation
D. Being - Becoming

High-level Importance

Unit 6

Questions 12–14

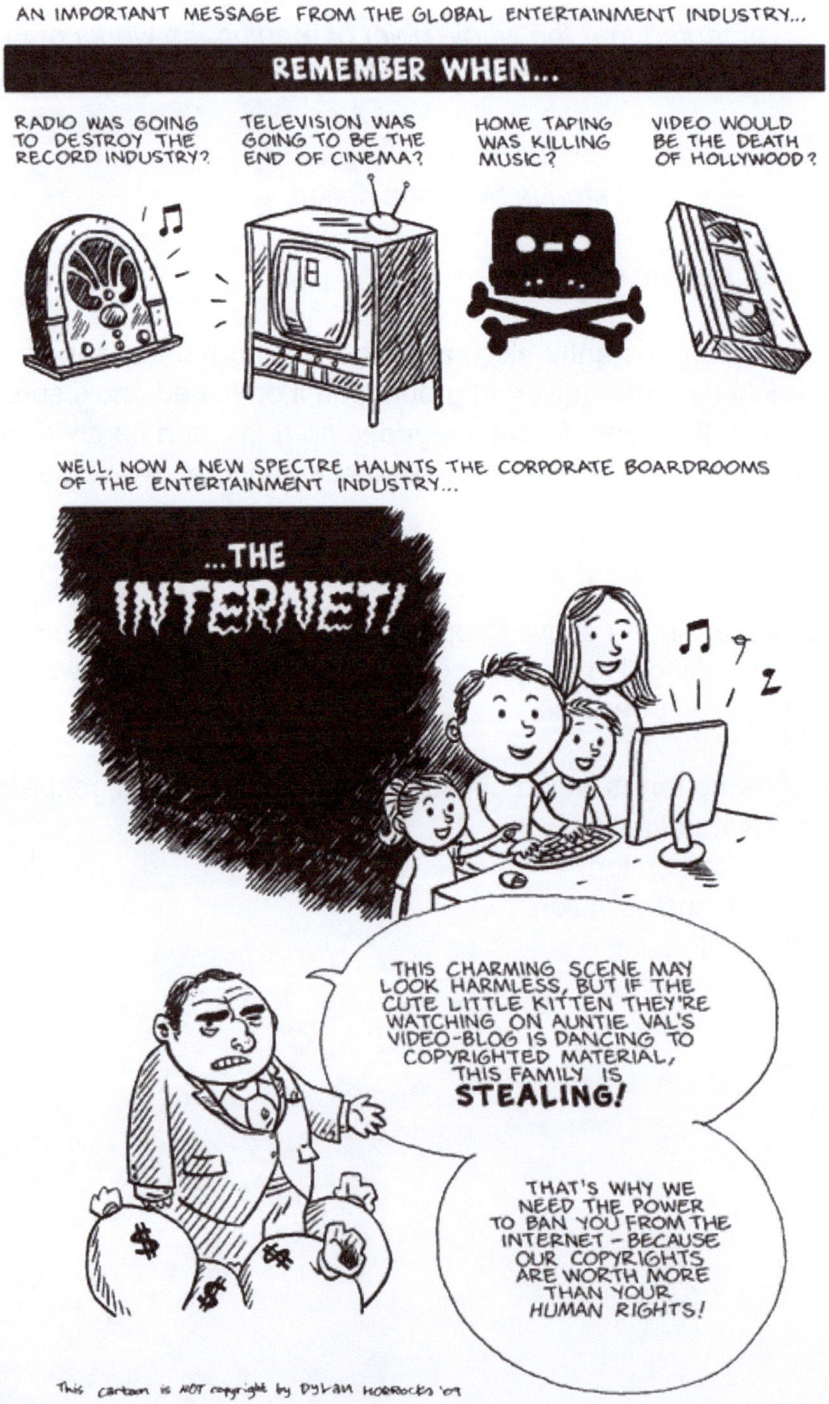

12. Which of the following groups of subjects would most adequately represent the contentious ideas presented within the cartoon?

- **A.** Popular Media, Hypertextuality, File-Sharing
- **B.** Intellectual Property, The Internet, Piracy
- **C.** Corporate Greed, Data Transfer, Representation
- **D.** Human Rights, Copyrights, Media

13. The humour of the cartoon mainly rests on:

- **A.** exaggeration.
- **B.** understatement.
- **C.** irony.
- **D.** cliché.

14. Presenting a historical comparison of the use of the internet to other forms of media is a form of argument that uses:

- **A.** definition.
- **B.** synthesis.
- **C.** induction.
- **D.** analogy.

Unit 7

Question 15

The following aphorism from the philosopher Nietzsche presents two seemingly asymmetrical concepts: chaos and creation. Given this odd pairing, one can make certain assumptions and inferences about Nietzsche's beliefs.

"Without chaos, how could one create a dancing star?"

15. Which of the following would not be a likely inference to be drawn from the statement by Nietzsche?

- **A.** Chaos is not viewed with negative connotations.
- **B.** Creativity and chaos are interlinked.
- **C.** Chaos is necessary for creation.
- **D.** Chaos precludes creativity.

If time remains, you may re-examine your work. If your allotted time (24 minutes) is complete, please proceed to the Answer Key.

3.7.1 Units 1–7 Answer Key and Worked Solutions

1.	C	**4.**	A	**7.**	D	**10.**	C	**13.**	C
2.	B	**5.**	D	**8.**	C	**11.**	B	**14.**	D
3.	C	**6.**	B	**9.**	D	**12.**	B	**15.**	D

1. A controlling metaphor can be thought of as a "main idea" type of question in relation to RHSS 3.5. In addition, this metaphor must be inferred based on the logic presented in the paragraph. (C) A metaphor can be inferred through the main idea within the first sentence. In describing the global economy, it can "be thought of as a complex international system, interlinked through the flow of goods, services, and information." The two terms "interlinked" and "flow" particularly stand out, indicating the metaphor of a "network." While (A) "medium" and (D) "hypertext" are certainly related, they do not encompass the complexity of the global economy as described in the passage. The metaphor of (B) "river" indicates the general notion of a flow and the possibilities of interlinkage, but is limited by one direction – that is, a river is linear while a complex network would have a flow in many different directions.

2. This is most certainly an "analysis of evidence" type of question in relation to RHSS 3.5. We are asked to make logical connections in relation to the evidence, as an example is being presented and extended. The (B) advent of information technologies would affect the spatial redistribution of labour and production – communication and the flow of information could be accomplished with relative ease on a global level. This line of thought follows logically from the first sentence in terms of a "flow of... information" aside from the outsourcing of labour and production in different countries. Since information is also a commodity, in many instances, (B) would be the correct choice. (A) can be ruled out as a non-sequitur. Although (C) "the rise of the minimum wage" and (D) "the displacement of labour due to economic factors" may have consequential effects on the rise of the global economy geographically, the more encompassing influence adhering to the idea of "global" would most certainly be the advances in technology and digital communications.

3. The answer is (C). (A) is easily excluded since an opinion is, by definition, subjective and therefore biased. (D) is also easily excluded as a savant is defined as one with unusually high mental capacity. (B) is more difficult as it could be argued that an atheist is devout to their beliefs about nothing as a subject. However, (C) is least oxymoronic because to be in a predicament means to be in a tough situation.

4. The poem identifies its subjects as belonging to the working class - for example, "housemaids". It paints a picture of a typical morning of the working class and says nothing about the upper class, so this eliminates option (C). Answer choice (D) is too literal and general to be the correct answer. On the other hand, the poem is specific in describing the depressed state of the working class: "damp souls", "twisted faces", a passerby with tears in the eyes and a smile that vanishes among the roofs - all suggesting sadness and dejection. "Basement kitchens", trampled or torn roads and "muddy skirts" depict a poor living condition. Nothing in the poem suggests (B) hope despite the miserable state of the subjects. In fact, the smile on one of the faces in the street is described as aimless and eventually vanishes, implying hopelessness. This leaves (A) as the best answer.

5. "Morning at the Window" presents a set of images of poverty, seen from the window of the speaker. It is not (A) an interpretation of someone's reflections on an experience. The poet, rather than expressing sympathies or feelings towards the working class' despondont state, chooses to merely describe various appearances and physical conditions of poverty. This eliminates options (B) and (C). The poet's impressions are then left for the individual reader to respond emotionally. This makes (D) the best answer.

6. Lines 15-19 provide the best clue in answering this question. The difference between "cyber crime" and "cyberterrorism" is often insubstantial, especially when the motive or the culprit of the crime is not clearly identified. Therefore, (B) is the correct choice, making (C) categorical and (D) well-defined the opposite and wrong answers. (A) Congruous means "in agreement". While both terms correspond to one another, the question asks what the nature of the difference between the two terms is - not what the nature of their relationship is.

7. The author is striving to be impartial by presenting definitions and clarifying concepts related to cyberterrorism. Hence, the correct answer is (D). The author is not (C) very opinionated since generalisations concerning the subject are supported with evidence through the use of examples and testimony rather than mere opinion. Similarly, while the author (A) may be possibly inferred to be against hacking and cyberterrorism, there are no calls to action for countermeasures nor is the language used emotionally-charged. The tone of writing may be rational, but it is neither disinterested nor (B) indifferent.

8. Even though (A), (B),& (D) are all true to some extent, the concepts do not necessarily relate to both of the ideas advanced in the question: the internet as a public utility within the context of terrorism; so by way of deduction, we find that (C) is the correct answer in that the internet shared by many, such as a public utility, is a likely, easily accessible, and vulnerable target to terrorist attacks. This is an "analysis of evidence" type of question as presented in RHSS 0.5. One makes assessments in a logical and deductive manner, by ruling out certain choices based on the evidence presented and its logical extension.

9. The correct choice is (D). Lines 5-6 state that "to qualify as cyberterrorism, an attack should result in violence against persons or property, or at least cause enough harm to generate fear". The examples provided in lines 23-26 indicate the extent of public damage and fear caused by cyber attacks in recent years. Options (A) and (C) require information outside of the passage in order to qualify the statements to be true or not. (B) is discussed as one of the main points in the passage, but this does not provide any evidence that will counter the idea that cyberterrorism is a myth.

10. The answer is (C). Although line 28 is non-specific, lines 29-30 go on to define an interdependency between both the private and public sectors. This is also implicit given the theme of interconnectivity throughout the stimulus. (A) is too specific and is implied in the other three options. (B) and (D) are also implied in (C).

11. (B) Aspiration – Perception is the correct answer. The first passage implies a "wish" (an aspiration into becoming something described in the story) that results in a sense of freedom and movement. Perception is quite correct in assessing the second passage since perception is interlinked with appearance. Answer (D) would be a close answer if the ratio was reversed to Becoming-Being to correspond to the order of the passages. There may or may not be an (A) initiation within the passage, but the term "naturalisation", albeit having connections to Nature – the tree, is vague, so this is not correct. (C) Alienation-Transformation is also very close, but the term "alienation" carries negative connotations. Undoubtedly, a transformation can be deduced to be occurring in the first passage but not in the second passage. This is a hybrid type of question, which presents abstract terms to define the main idea based on tone. So not only is the reader asked to relate an abstract term to a "main idea" type of question but also to review the "tone" of the passage by examining the dominant images.

12. All of the answer choices are at least partially correct. The most encompassing and specific in relation to the cartoon's contentions is (B). Through "an analysis of evidence" in assessing the main ideas presented within the material, this answer can be deduced. Again, we must determine what the most encompassing answer choice is while possessing the most explanatory power.

13. Options (B) and (D) can be readily eliminated among the answer choices. Nothing is (B) understated or (D) presented as an overused statement in the cartoon. It does seem like the rhetorical questions in the first set of images and the corporate character with the bags of money accusing the family to be stealing are (A) exaggerated assumptions. However, appreciating the humour of the cartoon requires looking at how the texts relate to the images. In the first set of images, 3 out of 4 technological representations do not appear to be threatening as described in the text. In the second set of images, the word "INTERNET" is written against a black, sinister-looking background and yet, the family viewing a video on the internet appears to be having fun. In the third image, while the corporate character labels the family's activity as stealing, he is portrayed to have a greedy agenda. The contrasts between what the texts are saying against what the pictures project indicate that the cartoon uses (C) irony to get its message across.

14. These comparisons are certainly an argument by (D) analogy by contrasting different forms of media throughout the years with the internet. (A) "Definition" is not correct because the internet is not being defined or interpreted as a specific media or medium. (B) An argument from "synthesis" would be a clash of ideas, in proper terms, dialectic and the result of this clash. This can be ruled out as well in relation to the cartoon. (C) "Induction" is close but not as encompassing as (D) analogy. As such, this question is "an analysis of evidence" type of question as referred to in RHSS 3.5.

15. All of the answers in relation to the Nietzsche quote can be inferred to some extent except (D), the correct choice. A certain degree of familiarity with vocabulary, particularly the term "precludes" is assumed and necessary to make the correct choice in (D). This phrase essentially would be antipodal – in opposition to the other assessments, meaning Chaos limits or rules out Creativity. This is an "inference" type of question, as presented in RHSS 3.5. We infer that all of the choices are correct, in relation, to the quote except for (D), which negates, instead of affirms a relation between the two: chaos and creativity.

3.7.2 Self-assessment

Consider your performance in the preceding short test and analysis:

- Did you finish answering all of the questions within 24 minutes?
- Were you able to answer most, if not all, of the questions correctly?

If you answered NO to at least one of these questions, then before proceeding to RHSS 3.8, we strongly advise that you access the Reading Speed and Comprehension Skill-builder Exercises in your online GAMSAT Humanities and Social Sciences lessons at GAMSAT-prep.com. Otherwise, you may start developing your reasoning skills for the Humanities and Social Sciences after your upcoming reading speed assessment.

3.7.3 Building Your Reading Speed and Comprehension Skills

The Gold Standard Reading Speed and Comprehension Skill-builder Exercises consist of at least five categories that each focusses on a particular type of text:

- Poems
- Excerpt From Novels
- Excerpts from Scientific Journals
- Philosophical Texts
- Visual Texts

Each exam category contains at least 10 separate timed Units that will test your speed and comprehension, and record your results. You may choose to attempt one Unit per category or just one category at a time in order to allow you to build your reading skills over time. Alternatively, you may attempt only those categories with which you have the most difficulty. Once you feel confident enough to tackle a particular type of passage in RHSS, you may begin attempting one of the related mini tests.

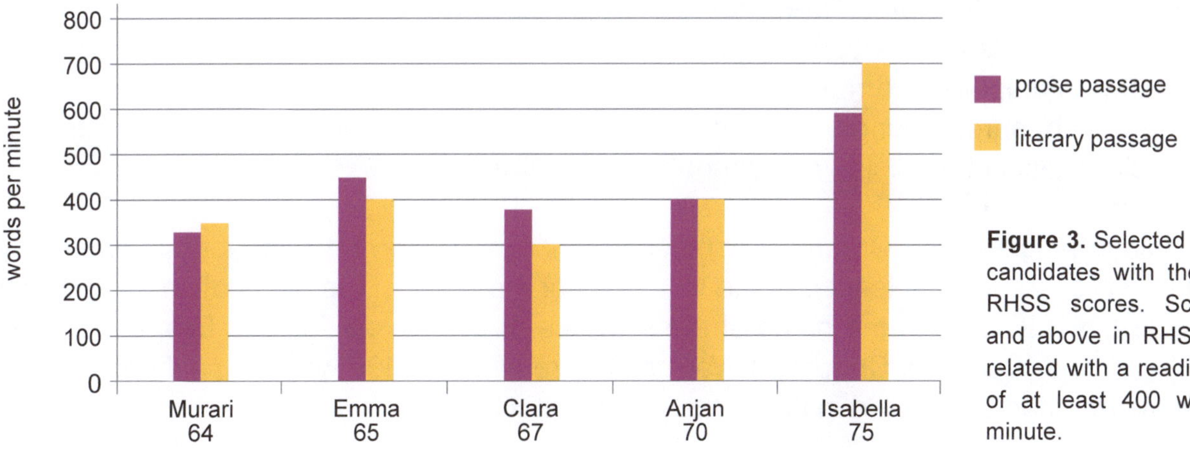

Figure 3. Selected GAMSAT candidates with their actual RHSS scores. Scoring 70 and above in RHSS is correlated with a reading speed of at least 400 words per minute.

Medium-level Importance

3.7.4 Reading Speed and Comprehension Test

If you already know your current reading speed, then you may choose to skip this section. Otherwise, the following test should be able to give you an idea of both your speed and comprehension rates. You will need a 'stopwatch' to perform this test. An online version with an automatic timer and instant score is also available when you log in to your GAMSAT-prep.com account.

Instructions:

1. *Turn on your 'stopwatch' as soon as you read the first word of the passage. Turn it off as you read the very last word in the text.*
2. *Note down the number of minutes (rounded to the nearest minute) in the box provided at the end of the passage.*
3. *Proceed to answer the short quiz to check your comprehension.*
4. *Calculate your reading speed by dividing the number of words of the passage by the number of minutes it took you to read.*
5. *Check your comprehension rate by dividing the total number of correct answers by the total number of questions. Multiply the result by 100.*

BEGIN ONLY WHEN TIMER IS READY.

As early as February 21, 1775, the Provincial Congress of Massachusetts appointed a committee to determine what medical supplies would be necessary should colonial troops be required to take the field. Three days later, the Congress voted to "make an inquiry where fifteen doctor's chests can be got, and on what terms"; and on March 7, it directed the committee of supplies "to make a draft in favour of Dr Joseph Warren and Dr Benjamin Church, for five hundred pounds, lawful money, to enable them to purchase such articles for the provincial chests of medicine as cannot be got on credit".

A unique ledger of the Greenleaf apothecary shop of Boston reveals that this pharmacy on April 4, 1775, supplied at least 5 of the 15 chests of medicines. The account, in the amount of just over £247, is listed in the name of the Province of the Massachusetts Bay, and shows that £51 was paid in cash by Dr Joseph Warren. The remaining £196 was not paid until August 10, after Warren had been killed in the Battle of Bunker Hill.

The 15 medicine chests, including presumably the five supplied by Greenleaf, were distributed on April 18—three at Sudbury and two each at Concord, Groton, Mendon, Stow, Worcester, and Lancaster. No record has been found to indicate whether or not the British discovered the medical chests at Concord, but, inasmuch as the patriots were warned of the British movement, it is very likely that the chests were among the supplies that were carried off and hidden. The British destroyed as much of the remainder as they could locate.

Total Reading Time: ____ *minutes*

1. What is the name of the pharmacy from which the committee purchased the medicine chests?

- **A.** Massachusetts
- **B.** The Apothecary Shop
- **C.** Concord
- **D.** Greenleaf

2. In whose account were the medical supplies listed?

- **A.** Dr Joseph Warren and Dr Benjamin Church
- **B.** Dr Joseph Warren
- **C.** Province of the Massachusetts Bay
- **D.** Greenleaf

3. Which amount would approximately represent the price of one medicine chest?

- **A.** £334
- **B.** £51
- **C.** £247
- **D.** £500

4. Three of the medicine chests were distributed at which location?

- **A.** Sudbury
- **B.** Concord
- **C.** Greenleaf
- **D.** Bunker Hill

5. The Provincial Congress of Massachusetts decided to canvass for 15 medicine chests on which date?
    A. February 21, 1775
    B. February 24, 1775
    C. March 7, 1775
    D. April 18, 1775

Answers

(P stands for Paragraph, S stands for Sentence; the corresponding numbers point to the paragraph number and the sentence within that paragraph.)

1. D P2 S1
2. C P2 S2
3. B P2 S2
4. A P3 S1
5. B P1 S2

The Provincial Congress of Massachusetts voted to "make an inquiry where fifteen doctor's chests can be got, and on what terms" three days after it appointed a committee for the medical supplies on February 21, 1775. February 21 plus 3 days makes February 24.

Score	Comprehension Rate
1	20%
2	40%
3	60%
4	80%
5	100%

What's my reading speed?

271 words / ____ minutes = _____ words per minute

Medium-level Importance

3.7.5 Interpreting Your Reading Speed

The slowest form of reading, 'mental reading', involves sounding out each word internally, as if you are actually reading to yourself (average: 250 words per minute, wpm). This is a form of subvocalisation, or silent speech.

'Auditory reading' can be optimised for GAMSAT Humanities and Social Sciences: Imagine hearing the read words (average: 450 wpm) but without subvocalisation. Note from our small cohort in the previous section, a reading speed of 300-400 wpm can result in very good Humanities and Social Sciences GAMSAT scores.

The fastest process is 'visual reading' which requires extensive practice and/or talent in order to maintain high levels of comprehension. This technique locks into understanding the meaning of the word, rather than sounding or hearing (average: 700 wpm).

3.8 GAMSAT Humanities and Social Sciences Mini Tests

We work hard to continually improve each new edition of the Gold Standard GAMSAT. Adding brand new content to textbooks is always exciting because of the prospect of enhancing the learning experience; however, it can be a bit hazardous because the content has not had the same level of exposure as 'older' content.

Nonetheless, we have tested our practice questions with hundreds of students prior to publication. As with the entire book, we have carefully edited the content. However, if you have any questions or concerns about any content in these new sections, please go to gamsat-prep.com/forum to find the Gold Standard GAMSAT Textbook Reasoning in Humanities and Social Sciences (RHSS; formerly: Section I) thread.

The following sections contain 6 mini tests that are grouped according to specific types of passages:

- Verbal Reasoning Exercise 1 (Humanities and Social Sciences)
- Verbal Reasoning Exercise 2 (Science-based Passages)
- Doctor-Patient Interaction Test
- Poetry Test
- Cartoon Test
- Graphs and Tables Test

The objective is to help build your Humanities and Social Sciences reasoning skills one area at a time. We strongly suggest that you ALWAYS time yourself for every practice test. Otherwise, you would be eliminating one of the major components of your preparation making it more difficult to get a top GAMSAT RHSS score. On the other hand, in the case that you are not pressured for time, do not assume that a specialty test is the same as a full-length exam. Just consider this experience as another step in your training.

At the end of each mini test, you should work through the answers and explanations. Keep notes of your wrong answers and then go back to the specific section(s) in this chapter, revising and analysing how you can still improve for your next attempts. Naturally, as you progress with your Humanities and Social Sciences studies, you should also consider full-length GAMSAT practice tests (i.e., Written Communication, RHSS and Sciences) including those from ACER and Gold Standard (the HEAPS exams).

Olympic athletes go to the gym to improve strength and fitness. The gym is not the sport. These mini tests are part of your Humanities and Social Sciences gym. Train well and it will be reflected in your performance.

3.8.1 Verbal Reasoning Exercise 1 (Humanities and Social Sciences)

The following is a sample mini test, aimed at developing your skills in reading and answering passages that contain arguments within the humanities or social science context. There are 7 Units with 40 questions. Choose the best answer for each question. You have 60 minutes. Please time yourself.

BEGIN ONLY WHEN TIMER IS READY.

Unit 1

Questions 1 - 6

Speech is so familiar a feature of daily life that we rarely pause to define it. It seems as natural to man as walking, and only less so than breathing. Yet it needs but a moment's reflection to convince us that this naturalness of speech is but an illusory feeling. The process of acquiring speech is, in sober fact, an utterly different sort of thing from the process of learning to walk. In the case of the latter function, culture, in other words, the traditional body of social usage is not seriously brought into play. The child is individually equipped, by the complex set of factors that we term biological heredity, to make all the needed muscular and nervous adjustments that result in walking.

Indeed, the very conformation of these muscles and of the appropriate parts of the nervous system may be said to be primarily adapted to the movements made in walking and in similar activities. In a very real sense the normal human being is predestined to walk, not because his elders will assist him to learn the art, but because his organism is prepared from birth, or even from the moment of conception, to take on all those expenditures of nervous energy and all those muscular adaptations that result in walking. To put it concisely, walking is an inherent, biological function of man.

Not so language. It is of course true that in a certain sense the individual is predestined to talk, but that is due entirely to the circumstance that he is born not merely in nature, but in the lap of a society that is certain, reasonably certain, to lead him to its traditions. Eliminate society and there is every reason to believe that he will learn to walk, if, indeed, he survives at all. But it is just as certain that he will never learn to talk, that is, to communicate ideas according to the traditional system of a particular society. Or, again, remove the newborn individual from the social environment into which he has come and transplant him to an utterly alien one. He will develop the art of walking in his new environment very much as he would have developed it in the old. But his speech will be completely at variance with the speech of his native environment.

Walking, then, is a general human activity that varies only within circumscribed limits as we pass from individual to individual. Its variability is involuntary and purposeless. Speech is a human activity that varies without assignable limit as we pass from social group to social group, because it is a purely historical heritage of the group, the product of long-continued social usage. It varies as all creative effort varies — not as consciously, perhaps, but none the less as truly as do the religions, the beliefs, the customs, and the arts of different peoples. Walking is an organic, an instinctive function (not, of course, itself an instinct); speech is a non-instinctive, acquired, "cultural" function.

- Excerpt from Edward Sapir, Language: An Introduction to the Study of Speech; 1921

1. What does the author **most likely** mean by the line "his speech will be completely at variance with the speech of his native environment" (paragraph 3)?
   - **A.** The child will speak a language that is not understood in his adoptive country.
   - **B.** The child will grow up speaking the language of his adoptive tribe or country.
   - **C.** The child's way of speaking will anger and antagonise people in his native country.
   - **D.** The child's way of speaking will shift between two sets of customs.

2. Which of the following pieces of information would support the author's claim that language is "the product of long-continued social usage"?
   - **A.** A discovery proved that languages across the world share some features in common, such as nouns, verbs and similar grammatical structures.
   - **B.** A deaf child raised without language input created her own gesture system that she used to form sentences.
   - **C.** Two neighbouring tribes could not effectively communicate with each other because their languages contained untranslatable concepts.
   - **D.** An extended family was found to have average overall intelligence and normal upbringings but were congenitally unable to learn a language.

3. Which contrasting concepts does the author suggest to be important in understanding the difference between walking and speech, respectively?
   A. Tradition vs innovation
   B. Reflex vs purpose
   C. Biology vs society
   D. Growth vs function

4. Which of the following does **not** follow the author's line of reasoning when he states that "speech is a human activity which varies without assignable limit"?
   A. Speech varies as we pass from one social group to another.
   B. Speech varies based on the cultural heritage of a social group.
   C. Speech varies based on a person's genetic capacity for complex grammar.
   D. Speech varies more than the instinctive sounds and cries made by animals.

5. The linguist Noam Chomsky has argued that young children learn language surprisingly quickly from a relatively small amount of input, and that a "consideration of [the] narrowly limited extent of the available data [that children are exposed to] leave[s] little hope that much of the structure of the language can be learned by an organism initially uninformed as to its general character".

   If true, this claim would:
   A. support the passage's argument because individual concepts are learned from a culture while a language's structure is innate.
   B. contradict the passage's argument because people do not learn a language as thoroughly as the author argues they do.
   C. support the passage's argument because babies are born without innate concepts for all the words they will eventually learn.
   D. contradict the passage's argument because people would have to be born with some innate knowledge of a language's natural character.

6. According to the author, speech is often mistakenly perceived as a natural function because:
   A. we rarely pause to define it.
   B. speech is socially acquired.
   C. it requires analysis to realise its purpose.
   D. speech is an effortless daily activity.

Unit 2

Questions 7 - 12

To the romantic poets, poetry was an instrument of emotion and feeling intended to reconnect man with the natural world, and in general, the poet was viewed as a person uniquely equipped to guide the layman to this reconnection.

Romanticism as a movement appeared following a period in history when great importance was put on scientific discovery and formal education. In the eyes of the romantic poets, mankind had become so swept up in the pursuit of knowledge and innovation that they had disconnected from both the natural world, and their deeper, natural selves. Though the philosophies of the individual poets differed, in general, romantic poetry focussed on and lauded primitivism and emotion while minimising (but not discounting) the importance of reason and logic. The ultimate goal of romantic poetry was the attainment of the sublime, the ultimate, transcendental connection with the natural self.

Samuel Taylor Coleridge, one of the pioneers of the Romantic Movement, believed that the creative imagination was the key to man achieving his connection to the sublime. This caused much difficulty though, as the source of creative imagination was impossible to trace and because creative inspiration was quite fickle. Coleridge struggled with this conundrum throughout his life but felt that as a poet and as one who understood the importance of the creative imagination, it was his right and responsibility to better mankind through his poetry. William Wordsworth was, along with Coleridge, another leader in the early Romantic Movement.

Wordsworth believed that beauty and inspiration were to be found in the most rudimentary and common things and was not something that could only be found in the high and lofty. It was the role of the poet to extract and explain that beauty. In his preface to "Lyrical Ballads," Wordsworth describes a poet as a man speaking to men, but ensures that he differentiates the poet as a man ". . . endowed with more lively sensibility, more enthusiasm and tenderness, who has a greater knowledge of human nature, and a more comprehensive soul, than are supposed to be common among mankind. . ." Thus, while rustic man could be privy to the sublime, it took the unique soul of a poet to make the sublime accessible to all. Like Coleridge, Wordsworth believed that creative imagination was the source of poetry and the avenue to the sublime. He was also of the belief that poetry was the result of the "spontaneous overflow of powerful feelings."

Percy Shelley not only believed that poets were charged with reconnecting man with nature, he believed poets were the "unacknowledged legislators of the world." He stated as much in "A Defence of Poetry," an essay in which he explained the importance of poetry in reconnecting man with feeling and emotion, and the importance of the poet as a person who could influence the course of mankind through this reconnection. However, unlike Coleridge and Wordsworth who sought out recognition and importance, Shelley recognised the role of the poet as one who affects mankind from the shadows of obscurity.

Though Coleridge, Wordsworth and Shelley may have differed in their individual poetic philosophies, the three poets, along with their Romantic colleagues, each strove to the same end. Each of these poets recognised great value in the natural feelings and emotions of man, and the connection sparked by man's place in the natural world. Each strove to capture and explain that connection through creative imagination and ultimately, through poetry.

7. The author suggests that the Romantic poets:
- **A.** attempted to attain the sublime and ultimate connection with one's natural self.
- **B.** believed they had the unique task of showing and reconnecting man with the natural world.
- **C.** thought science was diminishing man's creative imagination.
- **D.** were against Victorian morals and ways of thinking.

8. According to the passage, the problem with creative inspiration was that it was:
- **A.** something that could only be found in the high and lofty.
- **B.** to be found in the most unsophisticated things.
- **C.** impossible to trace.
- **D.** capricious.

9. Which of the following assertions is **not** made in the passage regarding Romanticism?
- **A.** It was a reaction to the burgeoning trend towards scientific and formal knowledge.
- **B.** It sought to reconnect man to his natural self through creative imagination.
- **C.** It challenged the use of reason and logic over emotion.
- **D.** It emphasised feelings and emotions as the key to man's reconnection with the natural world.

10. What is the author's purpose for writing the passage?

- **A.** To point out the differences in the Romantic poets and their philosophies
- **B.** To show that despite differences in their philosophies, the Romantics had the same end in mind
- **C.** To illustrate Romantic tendencies in juxtaposition to the idealism of the poets involved
- **D.** To capture the essence of Romanticism through the eyes of the various philosophers

11. The "sublime" is a concept that many critics and scholars would generally refer as indescribable but can take various forms such as a mountain, a landscape, a poem, a good meal, a heroic deed or a state of mind. Given the information on Coleridge and Wordsworth's Romantic principles, the sublime is considered:

- **A.** a form of spontaneous powerful emotion.
- **B.** attainable through creative imagination.
- **C.** ephemeral in the natural world.
- **D.** an inspired connection with one's natural self.

12. The more popular notion of the word "romantic" is that which is associated with love or strong affection and at times, irrationality. Which of the following assertions in the passage would be confused to be the same concept as those advanced by the Romantic Movement?

- **A.** The works of the Romantic poets such as the lyrical ballads often dealt with love.
- **B.** Romantic poets are also known for their typical temper and passion.
- **C.** The Romantic poets emphasised the importance of natural feelings and emotions in preference to reason and logic.
- **D.** Wordsworth claims that poetry is a result of the "spontaneous overflow of powerful feelings".

Unit 3

Questions 13 - 18

Gauguin's attitude toward art marked a break from the past and a beginning to modern art. He was from the start preoccupied with suggestion rather than description. Gauguin considered naturalism an error to be avoided, and he sought to render images in their purest, simplest and most primitive form. He wanted to portray the essence of things rather than the exterior form, which could only be achieved through simplification of the form. The beginning of his modern tradition lay in his rejection of Impressionism. He firmly believed throughout his life that "art is an abstraction" and that "this abstraction [must be derived] from nature while dreaming before it." One must think of the creation that will result rather than the model, and not try to render the model exactly as one sees it. Like all Post-Impressionist artists, he passed through an Impressionist phase but became quickly dissatisfied with the limitations of the style, and went on to discover a new style that had the directness and universality of a symbol and that concentrated on impressions, ideas and experiences. It was the birth of "Synthetism" or rather Synthetist-Symbolic, as Gauguin referred to it, using the term "symbolic" to indicate that the forms and patterns in his pictures were meant to suggest mental images or ideas and not simply to record a visual experience.

Symbolism flourished around the period of 1885 to 1910 and can be defined as the rejection of direct, literal representation in favour of evocation and suggestion. Painters tried to give a visual expression to emotional experiences, and therefore the movement was a reaction against the naturalistic aims of Impressionism. Satisfying the need for a more spiritual or emotional approach in art, Symbolism is characterised by the desire to seek refuge in a dream world of beauty and the belief that colour and line in themselves could express ideas. Stylistically, the tendency was towards flattened forms and broad areas of colour, and features of the movement were an intense religious feeling and an interest in subjects of death, disease, and sin.

Similarly, "Synthetism" involved the simplification of forms into large-scale patterns and the expressive purification of colours. Form and colour had to be simplified for the sake of expression. This style reacted against the "formlessness" of Impressionism and favoured painting subjectively and expressing one's ideas rather than relying on external objects as subject matters. It was characterised by areas of pure colours, very defined contours, an emphasis on pattern and decorative qualities, and a relative absence of shadows.

Gauguin's new art form merged these two movements and succeeded in freeing colour, form, and line, bringing it to express the artists' emotions, sensibilities, and personal experiences of the world around them. His style created a break with the old tradition of descriptive naturalism and favoured the synthesis of observation and imagination. Gauguin sustained that forms are not discovered in nature but in one's wild imagination, and it was in himself that he searched rather than in his surroundings. For this reason, he scorned the Impressionists for their lack of imagination and their mere scientific reasoning. Furthermore, Gauguin used colour unnaturalistically for its decorative or emotional effect and reintroduced emphatic outlines. "Synthetism" signified for him that the forms of his pictures were constructed from symbolic patterns of colour and linear rhythms and were not mere scientific reproductions of what is seen by the eye.

13. Based on passage information, which of the following can you infer to be among the principles of Impressionism?

A. Representing idealised versions of reality as they exist in the artist's mind
B. Representing reality using technical tools such as photography to capture its appearance
C. Representing the outward forms of things exactly as they appear to the naked eye
D. Representing the feelings derived from an experience through vibrant colours and lines

14. According to passage information, what do Symbolism and Impressionism have in common?

A. Both saw ideas as crucial to the impact of a work.
B. Both focused on representing nature rather than man-made objects.
C. Both considered the artist's subjective experience to be a key element to the work.
D. Both thought art needed to express the idiosyncratic nature of the artist rather than pleasing society.

15. Which of the following hypothetical pieces of evidence would diminish the author's claims about the importance of Gauguin?

A. Evidence that Gauguin's style of painting was based on work by van Gogh and other painters active during the 1870s and 80s
B. Evidence that both Gauguin and the Impressionists rejected the more formal and conventional realism of the early 1800s
C. Photographic evidence that some of Gauguin's works bear no apparent resemblance to the landscape they were supposedly based on
D. Evidence that the Impressionists' works were considered just as shocking and revolutionary in their time as Gauguin's work would later be

High-level Importance

16. Based on passage information, which of these quotes from fellow painters would Gauguin **least likely** agree?

- **A.** "Treat nature in terms of the cylinder, the sphere, and the cone." *(Paul Cezanne)*
- **B.** "Painting is a blind man's profession. He paints not what he sees, but what he feels, what he tells himself about what he has seen." *(Pablo Picasso)*
- **C.** "Paintings have a life of their own that derives from the painter's soul." *(Vincent van Gogh)*
- **D.** "There is only one true thing: instantly paint what you see. When you've got it, you've got it. When you haven't, you begin again." *(Édouard Manet)*

17. According to the passage, Gauguin rejected Impressionism for a number of reasons. Which of the following **cannot** be inferred to have been a motive of this rejection?

- **A.** Lack of flexibility within the style of Impressionism
- **B.** Lack of intense feelings and emotions in Impressionism
- **C.** Lack of beauty in Impressionism
- **D.** Lack of imagination in Impressionism

18. Elsewhere, it is said that Japanese art influenced Gauguin's work. Given the passage discussion of Synthetist-Symbolism, which of these features of Japanese painting can be reasonably assumed to characterise Gauguin's art form?

- **A.** Use of fluid curved lines
- **B.** Use of animals and landscapes as subjects
- **C.** Use of narrative elements to express ideas
- **D.** Use of strong colours and compositional freedom

Unit 4

Questions 19 - 25

Human conduct and belief are now undergoing transformations profounder and more disturbing than any since the appearance of wealth and philosophy put an end to the traditional religion of the Greeks.

It is the age of Socrates again: our moral life is threatened, and our intellectual life is quickened and enlarged by the disintegration of ancient customs and beliefs. Everything is new and experimental in our ideas and our actions; nothing is established or certain any more. The rate, complexity, and variety of change in our time are without precedent, even in Periclean days; all forms about us are altered, from the tools that complicate our toil, and the wheels that whirl us restlessly about the earth, to the innovations in our sexual relationships and the hard disillusionment of our souls.

The passage from agriculture to industry, from the village to the town, and from the town to the city has elevated science, debased art, liberated thought, ended monarchy and aristocracy, generated democracy and socialism, emancipated woman, disrupted marriage, broken down the old moral code, destroyed asceticism with luxuries, replaced Puritanism with Epicureanism, exalted excitement above content, made war less frequent and more terrible, taken from us many of our most cherished religious beliefs and given us a mechanical and fatalistic philosophy of life. All things flow, and we seek some mooring and stability in the flux.

In every developing civilisation, a period comes when old instincts and habits prove inadequate to altered stimuli, and ancient institutions and moralities crack like hampering shells under the obstinate growth of life. In one sphere after another, now that we have left the farm and the home for the factory, the office and the world, spontaneous and "natural" modes of order and response break down, and intellect chaotically experiments to replace with conscious guidance the ancestral readiness and simplicity of impulse and wonted ways. Everything must be thought out, from the artificial "formula" with which we feed our children, and the "calories" and "vitamins" of our muddled dietitians, to the bewildered efforts of a revolutionary government to direct and coordinate all the haphazard processes of trade. We are like a man who cannot walk without thinking of his legs, or like a player who must analyse every move and stroke as he plays. The happy unity of instinct is gone from us, and we flounder in a sea of doubt; amidst unprecedented knowledge and power, we are uncertain of our purposes, values and goals.

From this confusion, the one escape worthy of a mature mind is to rise out of the moment and the part and contemplate the whole. What we have lost above all is total perspective. Life seems too intricate and mobile for us to grasp its unity and significance; we cease to be citizens and become only individuals; we have no purposes that look beyond our death; we are fragments of men, and nothing more.

No one (except Spengler) dares today to survey life in its entirety; analysis leaps and synthesis lags; we fear the experts in every field and keep ourselves, for safety's sake, lashed to our narrow specialties. Everyone knows his part, but is ignorant of its meaning in the play. Life itself grows meaningless and becomes empty just when it seemed most full.

Let us put aside our fear of inevitable error, and survey all those problems of our state, trying to see each part and puzzle in the light of the whole. We shall define philosophy as "total perspective," as mind overspreading life and forging chaos into unity. Perhaps philosophy will give us, if we are faithful to it, a healing unity of soul. We are so slovenly and self-contradictory in our thinking; it may be that we shall clarify ourselves and pull ourselves together into consistency and be ashamed to harbour contradictory desires or beliefs. And through this unity of mind may come that unity of purpose and character which makes a personality and lends some order and dignity to our existence. Philosophy is harmonised knowledge making a harmonious life; it is the self-discipline which lifts us to security and freedom. Knowledge is power, but only wisdom is liberty.

Our culture is superficial today, and our knowledge dangerous, because we are rich in mechanisms and poor in purposes. The balance of mind which once came of a warm religious faith is gone; science has taken from us the supernatural bases of our morality and all the world seems consumed in a disorderly individualism that reflects the chaotic fragmentation of our character.

We move about the earth with unprecedented speed, but we do not know, and have not thought, where we are going, or whether we shall find any happiness there for our harassed souls. We are being destroyed by our knowledge, which has made us drunk with our power. And we shall not be saved without wisdom.

19. What could be inferred as the best title for this passage?

- **A.** What is Philosophy?
- **B.** The Age of Uncertainty
- **C.** The Dualities of Wisdom
- **D.** How We can Progress

20. The tone of the author is:

- **A.** bleak.
- **B.** hopeful.
- **C.** existential.
- **D.** cautious.

21. Which of the following statements would **most likely** contradict the author's thesis?

- **A.** Inconsistency is the key to flexibility.
- **B.** Values and morals are essentially socially-constructed.
- **C.** A given culture's development of wisdom in relation to the world's fragmentation is determined by symbolic behaviour.
- **D.** There is progress in technology in relation to a higher sense of spiritual development.

22. How does the author define philosophy?

I. As a "total perspective"
II. As mind overspreading life and forging chaos into unity
III. As the essential balance between mind and matter

A. I only
B. II only
C. I and II
D. I, II, and III

23. Based on passage information, philosophy is based according to which of the following notions?

A. A synthesis of opposites
B. A struggle for progress
C. A reaching for goodness
D. Harmony

24. In the passage, the author assigns knowledge and wisdom to particular representations. Which of the following best exemplifies this ratio?

A. Power-Liberty
B. Essence-Existence
C. Being-Becoming
D. Static-Active

25. The author claims that the movement from agriculture to industry gave people a fatalistic and mechanical view of life. Within the post-industrial age we currently live in, the movement to the digital world has given people a view of life, which is:

A. disconnected and shallow.
B. connected and hopeful.
C. simultaneously interconnected yet disassociated.
D. a network of linear lines of information affecting humanity globally.

Unit 5

Questions 26 - 32

The Sick Rose by William Blake

O Rose thou art sick.
The invisible worm,
That flies in the night
In the howling storm:
Has found out thy bed
Of crimson joy:
And his dark secret love
Does thy life destroy.

Here the title encapsulates the essential dynamic of the poem. The rose is an archetypal symbol, which means that it has been seized on by all cultures which have known roses as symbolising very much the same range of human experience, and is spontaneously recognised as doing so even by those who do not know what a symbol is.

Archetypes contain the ability to release a certain range of meanings with peculiar depth and power. Things become symbols because of characteristics evident in ordinary life, and these remain the primary elements in the symbol however much it might have been elaborated in the literary tradition. We are all aware of the rose as a queen of flowers, beautiful, rich in colour (especially the red rose), heady in perfume, sensuous in texture, incurved, enfolding erotic promise. The rose activates all the senses like the body of a desired woman. Rose metaphors are part of our common language. Rosy cheeks signify health; rosy lips are asking to be kissed. Few men have never sent a woman a bunch of red roses; and even when there is no verbal message, the woman has no difficulty knowing what that means. Burns wrote: 'My love is like a red, red, rose'. In giving a woman a red rose, a man is giving her an image of herself, or herself as he would wish her to be, rich with sexual passion.

As a primary female sexual symbol, the rose in the ancient world was attributed to Aphrodite/Venus, goddess of sexual love. The book which distilled and defined the courtly love invented by the medieval troubadours was called the Roman de la Rose, where the rose symbolises a woman's awakening to sexual love.

If we add together all the associations of the word rose, those we supply from our own experience, those common in our culture, and those we happen to be familiar with in the literary tradition, we have a very strong sense of youth, health, beauty and joy, of the feminine at its most desirable, of vitality and creativity, of the gratification of erotic desires. The last adjective we anticipate is 'sick'. Sickness, disease, corruption, are not only contrary to all the primary meanings of 'rose' but strike us as a violation of them, a sacrilege. The two words cancel each other out, leaving a void, a chaos. The title enacts linguistically the degradation of the rose the poem then dramatises. Blake was by no means the first poet to exploit this shock effect. In *A Midsummer Night's Dream* Shakespeare, needing to convey what happens when the natural progression of the seasons is violated and Great Creating Nature made sterile, writes: 'heavy-headed frosts / Fall in the fresh lap of the crimson rose'. And in Lycidas Milton wrote 'as killing as the canker to the rose'.

The poets Blake was most familiar with and most respected were Shakespeare and Milton, and he expected his readers to know them well. 'The Sick Rose' draws so heavily on both of them that it can hardly be read, or loses half its force, if the reader is unaware of the power and quite specific meanings flowing into this poem from *Twelfth Night*, *Hamlet* and *Paradise Lost*.

In Book IX of *Paradise Lost*, Satan, having crossed the howling storm of chaos, 'with meditated guile' flies 'as a mist by night' into Eden, where he enters the serpent, the fittest creature to communicate his 'dark suggestions' to Eve. (The first meaning of 'worm' in the Oxford English Dictionary is 'serpent, snake, dragon'.) Satan views Eve " . . . so thick the roses bushing round about her glowed" to which she is compared to, with a "storm so nigh" given as a background context from where Satan has come from. His avowed purpose is 'all pleasure to destroy' since he has lost his own capacity for joy. When Eve tells Adam what has happened, he describes her as 'deflowered': From his slack hand the garland wreathed for Eve, down dropped, and all the faded roses shed.

Nakedness and sex become for both of them a cause for shame, which they had never known before. This story, with its memorable imagery of the invisible tempter flying through a howling storm, becoming a worm, and desecrating the joy of the marriage bed for both man and woman, clearly looms behind 'The Sick Rose' and feeds it with potent suggestions. These suggestions mingle with others from Shakespeare. The worm which destroys the beauty of a young woman must remind us of Viola's story of an imaginary sister: She never told her love, But let concealment, like a worm i' the bud, Feed on her damask cheek: she pin'd in thought. The examples lend their credence that "The Sick Rose" is remarkably influenced by Milton and Shakespeare.

High-level Importance

26. Given that the rose is an archetype recognised by all cultures as a symbol, it can be inferred that:

A. poetry, as an aspect of culture, is an archetype which is created through symbolisation.
B. the archetype is understood through language and interpretation of the referent.
C. things are symbolised through evidentiary and ordinary characteristics representing the same elements.
D. symbols are a generalised and universal aspect of all cultures as evidenced through archetypes.

27. By linking the contrary meanings of "sick and rose," the poem itself displays:

A. an oxymoron throwing the reader into an abyss of chaos.
B. a juxtaposition between romantic and destructive imagery.
C. a tonality and effect which contradict each other linguistically.
D. an explosion of multiple meanings and effects on the reader.

28. The author's attitude towards archetypes can be characterised as:

A. telescopic.
B. critical.
C. focussed.
D. encompassing.

29. The commentator refers to Milton in *Paradise Lost* in order to emphasise the beginning of:

A. sin.
B. the fall from Grace.
C. shame.
D. dualism.

30. Within the passage, it can be reasonably noted that the meaning of archetypes in culture have:

A. profound reflections of man's common consciousness.
B. associations with a certain range of intention.
C. influences on the literary tradition.
D. interrelations with linguistic structures.

31. Based on the author's discussions, if a reader is unfamiliar with Blake's allusions to Milton and Shakespeare:
- **A.** the rose will be overlooked as an essential archetype in the poem.
- **B.** the meaning of the poem loses half its force and power.
- **C.** the meaning of the poem will be lost in superficial interpretation.
- **D.** the worm will be misinterpreted within the scope of the poem's imagery.

32. The characterisation of Blake's poem with Milton can be reasonably described as:
- **A.** redundant.
- **B.** irrevocable.
- **C.** inharmonious.
- **D.** uncanny.

Unit 6

Questions 33 - 37

The "Theatre of the Absurd" is a term coined by Hungarian-born critic Martin Esslin, who made it the title of his 1962 book on the subject. The term refers to a particular type of play which first became popular during the 1950s and 1960s and which presented on stage the philosophy articulated by French philosopher Albert Camus in his 1942 essay, "The Myth of Sisyphus", in which he defines the human condition as basically meaningless. Camus argued that humanity had to resign itself to recognising that a fully satisfying rational explanation of the universe was beyond its reach; in that sense, the world must ultimately be seen as absurd.

Esslin regarded the term "Theatre of the Absurd" merely as a "device" by which he meant to bring attention to certain fundamental traits discernible in the works of a range of playwrights. The playwrights loosely grouped under the label of the absurd attempt to convey their sense of bewilderment, anxiety, and wonder in the face of an inexplicable universe. According to Esslin, the five defining playwrights of the movement are Eugène Ionesco, Samuel Beckett, Jean Genet, Arthur Adamov, and Harold Pinter, although these writers were not always comfortable with the label and sometimes preferred to use terms such as "Anti-Theatre" or "New Theatre". Other playwrights associated with this type of theatre include Tom Stoppard, Arthur Kopit, Friedrich Dürrenmatt, Fernando Arrabal, Edward Albee, N.F. Simpson, Boris Vian, Peter Weiss, Vaclav Havel, and Jean Tardieu. The most famous, and most controversial, absurdist play is probably Samuel Beckett's *Waiting for Godot.* The characters of the play are strange caricatures who have difficulty communicating the simplest of concepts to one another as they bide their time awaiting the arrival of Godot. The language they use is often ludicrous, and following the cyclical pattern, the play seems to end in precisely the same condition it began, with no real change having occurred. In fact, it is sometimes referred to as "the play where nothing happens." Its detractors count this a fatal flaw and often turn red in the face fomenting on its inadequacies. It is mere gibberish, they cry, eyes nearly bulging out of their head - a prank on the audience disguised as a play. The plays supporters, on the other hand, describe it is an accurate parable on the human condition in which "the more things change, the more they are the same." Change, they argue, is only an illusion. In 1955, the famous character actor Robert Morley predicted that the success of *Waiting for Godot* meant "the end of theatre as we know it." His generation may have gloomily accepted this prediction, but the younger generation embraced it. They were ready for something new - something that would move beyond the old stereotypes and reflect their increasingly complex understanding of existence.

Whereas traditional theatre attempts to create a photographic representation of life as we see it, the Theatre of the Absurd aims to create a ritual-like, mythological, archetypal, allegorical vision, closely related to the world of dreams. The focal point of these dreams is often man's fundamental bewilderment and confusion, stemming from the fact that he has no answers to the basic existential questions: why we are alive, why we have to die, why there is injustice and suffering. Ionesco defined the absurdist everyman as "Cut off from his religious, metaphysical, and transcendental roots … lost; all his actions become senseless, absurd, useless." The Theatre of the Absurd, in a sense, attempts to reestablish man's communion with the universe. Dr. Jan Culik writes, "Absurd Theatre can be seen as an attempt to restore the importance of myth and ritual to our age, by making man aware of the ultimate realities of his condition, by instilling in him again the lost sense of cosmic wonder and primaeval anguish. The Absurd Theatre hopes to achieve this by shocking man out of an existence that has become trite, mechanical and complacent. It is felt that there is mystical experience in confronting the limits of human condition."

- Adapted from J. Crabb, Theatre of the Absurd; 2006

33. The author's tone in paragraph 2 discussing critics of Waiting for Godot can be described as:

A. analytical.
B. persuasive.
C. mocking.
D. definitional.

34. One can infer from passage information that "Theatre of the Absurd" plays:

I. contain naturalistic dialogue based on the rhythms of speech.
II. involve plots based on those of classical myths.
III. alters viewers' perceptions of reality after they leave the theatre.

A. I and III
B. I, II, and III
C. I only
D. III only

35. Based on passage information, it can be inferred that in Samuell Beckett's play *Waiting for Godot*:

A. the characters are mouthpieces for the author in accurately describing the absurdity of existence.
B. the concept of waiting is given cosmic significance as both characters and audience wait for something that will never occur.
C. the author provides an ambivalent statement on human existence because while the characters' lives do not improve, they also do not get any worse.
D. Becket caricatures the ridiculous and shallow people of his time through the stilted words and actions of the characters.

36. Based on passage information, the playwrights under discussion in this passage used absurdity in order to:

A. make viewers newly aware of the absurdity of human life.
B. shock viewers who believed all theatre should reflect life realistically.
C. provide a respite from the humdrum of normal life.
D. express their real selves and the uniquely strange way they experienced life.

37. The author implies that the "Theatre of the Absurd" could be considered:

A. a branch of realism.
B. a step in the evolution toward today's artistic forms.
C. a genre of literature.
D. a template for producing artistic works.

Unit 7

Questions 38 - 40

At the present time, when women are beginning to take part in the affairs of the world, it is still a world that belongs to men – they have no doubt of it at all and women have scarcely any. To decline to be the Other, to refuse to be a party to the deal – this would be for women to renounce all the advantages conferred upon them by their alliance with the superior caste. Man-the-sovereign will provide woman-the-liege with material protection and will undertake the moral justification of her existence; thus she can evade at once both economic risk and the metaphysical risk of a liberty in which ends and aims must be contrived without assistance. Indeed, along with the ethical urge of each individual to affirm his subjective existence, there is also the temptation to forgo liberty and become a thing. This is an inauspicious road, for he who takes it – passive, lost, ruined – becomes henceforth the creature of another's will, frustrated in his transcendence and deprived of every value. But it is an easy road; on it, one avoids the strain involved in undertaking an authentic existence. When man makes of woman the Other, he may, then, expect to manifest deep-seated tendencies towards complicity. Thus, woman may fail to lay claim to the status of subject because she lacks definite resources, because she feels the necessary bond that ties her to man regardless of reciprocity, and because she is often very well pleased with her role as the Other.

- Excerpt from Simone de Beauvoir, Woman as Other; 1949

38. According to the author, the relationship that transpires between man and woman is that of:

A. a master to his slave.
B. a communal partnership.
C. a provider and his dependent.
D. a conspiracy.

39. The author suggests that the roles of men and women are dictated by:

A. survival needs.
B. male orientation.
C. social preconditions.
D. personal motives.

40. According to the author, the woman considers herself as:

A. a dependent of man.
B. a willing subordinate of man.
C. an insecure social being.
D. man's moral responsibility.

If time remains, you may re-examine your work. If your allotted time (60 minutes) is complete, please proceed to the Answer Key.

3.8.2 Verbal Reasoning Exercise 1 (Humanities and Social Sciences) Answer Key and Worked Solutions

1.	B	**9.**	C	**17.**	C	**25.**	C	**33.**	C
2.	C	**10.**	B	**18.**	D	**26.**	C	**34.**	D
3.	C	**11.**	B	**19.**	A	**27.**	B	**35.**	B
4.	C	**12.**	C	**20.**	C	**28.**	D	**36.**	A
5.	D	**13.**	C	**21.**	D	**29.**	C	**37.**	C
6.	D	**14.**	C	**22.**	C	**30.**	A	**38.**	C
7.	B	**15.**	A	**23.**	D	**31.**	B	**39.**	C
8.	D	**16.**	D	**24.**	A	**32.**	D	**40.**	B

1. **Correct Answer: B**

This question asks what the author is claiming in his hypothetical scenario of an infant being transported to a different land. Sapir argues that the child would learn to walk in the same way regardless of which environment he was brought up in, but will learn a language in a specific way in the context of his new culture (rather than his native one). Thus he will speak the language of the adoptive land rather than the native one. This rules out answer choice (A). The example given in option (B) concerns someone who is transported to an adoptive land at a young age and thus learns its language. Therefore, it is the correct answer.

The context of this sentence assumes that the child has been permanently "transplanted" to the new social environment, so his language may no longer bear resemblance to his original (i.e., native) environment. The paragraph does not imply that when this happens, this will (C) anger the people in his native country. Likewise, the author uses "at variance" to suggest deep-seated difference rather than (D) changes or shifts in spoken language over time.

2. **Correct Answer: C**

To answer this question, you must determine which hypothetical facts would support or weaken the passage's main argument, which states that language varies without limit - that languages are "a purely historical heritage of the group, the product of long-continued social usage". Thus the discovery that some languages contain culture-specific concepts and are vastly different would support the passage's claims. This makes (C) the best option.

(A) This discovery would weaken the claim that languages vary "without limit".

(B) The author states that language is not an innate function and that an individual learns to speak because "he is born... in the lap of a society that is certain, reasonably certain, to lead him to its traditions." Thus if a discovery was made that a person learned a language without being taught society's traditions of speech, this argument would weaken his claims.

(D) The fact that a family all suffered from a congenital condition would suggest it is hereditary. If people had enough intelligence to learn other information but were prevented from learning language by a hereditary condition, this would suggest that language has a biological aspect.

3. **Correct Answer: C**

This question asks what dichotomies are mentioned in the passage as separating speech from other human activities such as walking. Several instances in the excerpt emphasise biological development as a factor for walking as opposed to society's influence on an individual's speech development. This makes (C) the best answer.

(A) The author does mention tradition in the context of a culture, but it neither mentions innovation nor suggests that it is important to understanding speech.

(B) The author states that walking would eventually happen as a natural reflex but does not omphasise purpose as a factor in developing speech.

(D) The author states that walking will occur as an individual grows "if he survives at all". However, the author refers to walking and talking as - both - functions albeit instinctive and acquired, respectively.

4. **Correct Answer: C**

This question requires you to think about the implications of one of the author's main arguments. The claim that (C) speech varies based on genetics does not follow from the author's reasoning since a function that is genetically-based is innate and thus places a built-in limitation on how much it could vary (just as with human walking and running abilities).

(A) The author's notion of variation based on cultural differences means speech would vary between groups.

(B) The author states that "society... is certain, reasonably certain, to lead [a speaker] to its traditions" - in other words, the cultural heritage of the social group to which he belongs.

(D) The author states that speech varies according to culture; since animals lack culture, their communicative sounds would not vary as much.

5. **Correct Answer: D**

This question necessitates that you to think about the implications of a claim by another author (Chomsky) to the argument presented by the passage's author. Chomsky is saying that babies do not have access to as much data as they would need to learn an entire language from scratch. From the fact that people do eventually learn to speak their native languages, we can infer that people acquire language using not just cultural learning but some pre-existing information about a language's general character. This would contradict Sapir's claim that language is not an "inherent, biological function of man". The correct answer is (D).

(A) The passage never discusses a distinction between content and structure or suggests that any aspect of language is innate.

(B) Neither Chomsky nor Sapir expressed true doubt that people learn a language thoroughly.

(C) The quote from Chomsky suggests that young children are born with innate information about a language's general character in order to learn the structure of a language. This contradicts rather than supports Sapir's argument that language is only acquired through culture and social tradition, not by pre-existing information.

6. **Correct Answer: D**

Answering this question requires understanding the context of the author's premise that the "naturalness of speech is but an illusory feeling". This can be found in the first 3 sentences of the passage, which explains that speech, being part of our daily activities, is too familiar a function as breathing that we talk without requiring a deliberate effort to do so. This is the main reason why the author believes we often mistake speech as a natural function when it is actually socially acquired. The best option is (D).

(A) The author does state, "Speech is so familiar a feature of daily life that we rarely pause to define it." However, this is only part of his explanation as to the main reason why he deems speech to be an unnatural function. Also, please note that answer choices that are almost verbatim of a line from the passage are frequently used as a decoy and are thus incorrect.

(B) This is a true statement. The passage indeed argues that speech is acquired through one's social environment. However, this does not really answer the question, does it? (*See* RHSS 3.2.5 Technique Number 5.)

(C) The author says that "it needs but a moment's reflection" to realise that speech is not a natural function but does not mention about needing to realise the purpose of talking.

7. **Correct Answer: B**

This question requires differentiating the author's view and statements about the Romantic poets in general, from those of the three Romantic poets referred in the passage:

"To the romantic poets, poetry was an instrument of emotion and feeling intended to reconnect man with the natural world, and in general the poet was viewed as a person uniquely equipped to guide the layman to this reconnection." (P1)

"Each of these poets recognised great value in the natural feelings and emotions of man, and the connection sparked by man's place in the natural world. Each strove to capture and explain that connection through creative imagination and ultimately, through poetry." (Last paragraph)

(A) This option is a misreading of the information found in the last sentence of Paragraph 2 pertaining to the goal of Romantic poetry - not poets.

(C) This is another misreading of the idea that "In the eyes of the romantic poets, mankind had become so swept up in the pursuit of knowledge and innovation that they had disconnected from both the natural world, and their deeper, natural selves." The Romantic poets saw the scientific discoveries diminishing man's connection with the natural selves and the world – not creative imagination. In fact, they also valued reason and logic as indicated in P2 S3:

"Though the philosophies of the individual poets differed, in general romantic poetry focussed on and lauded primitivism and emotion while minimising (but not discounting) the importance of reason and logic."

(D) This answer is an anachronism, i.e., the Victorian era comes after the Romantic age temporally.

8. **Correct Answer: D**

This is another question that calls for differentiating the concepts and perspectives presented in the passage. The trick in this question lies in the use of the terms "creative inspiration" and "creative imagination," which can get incorrectly interchanged and thus easily misinterpreted because they are being used in various details and concepts.

The answer can be readily found in P3 S2:

"This caused much difficulty though, as the source of creative imagination was impossible to trace and because creative inspiration was quite fickle."

This opposes Wordsworth's belief that inspiration is derived from the most basic and simplest of things:

"Wordsworth believed that beauty and inspiration were to be found in the most rudimentary and common things and was not something that could only be found in the high and lofty." (P4 S1)

(A) This is in contradiction to Wordsworth's view of beauty and inspiration.

(B) The passage does not imply that this is a problem of creative inspiration, as indicated in P4 S1.

(C) This refers to creative imagination - not inspiration.

9. **Correct Answer: C**

Although Romanticism as a movement was formed during the height of scientific discoveries, it did not essentially (C) challenge the use of reason and logic, but rather of man's tendency to be consumed by "the pursuit of knowledge and innovation" as indicated in P2:

"In the eyes of the romantic poets, mankind had become so swept up in the pursuit of knowledge and innovation that they had disconnected from both the natural world, and their deeper, natural selves. Though the philosophies of the individual poets differed, in general romantic poetry focussed on and lauded primitivism and emotion while minimising (but not discounting) the importance of reason and logic."

(A) The Romantic movement is thus in response, indeed, (though not necessarily a challenge) to the scientific and formal knowledge at that time. (P2 S2)

(B) This is supported in the last sentence of Paragraph 2 and the last paragraph. Beliefs of the three Romantic poets mentioned also emphasise this idea. (P3 S1, P4 S5, P5 S2)

(D) This is clearly stated in the second sentence of the last paragraph.

10. Correct Answer: B

The essay does not focus on just (A) differences, so this option can be ruled out. Nor does the essay focus on (D) "philosophers". (C) mentions "tendencies," which is ambiguous as this statement neither specifies poetic tendencies nor does the passage involve "juxtaposition" which implies a difference. This leaves (B) as the most inclusive of the answer choices.

11. Correct Answer: B

The question specifies an answer that involves identifying a common view between Coleridge and Wordsworth on to the "sublime". These can be found in the following lines:

"Samuel Taylor Coleridge, one of the pioneers of the Romantic Movement, believed that the creative imagination was the key to man achieving his connection to the sublime." (P3 S1)

"Like Coleridge, Wordsworth believed that creative imagination was the source of poetry and the avenue to the sublime." (P4 S5)

The rest are decoys that are meant to sound like commonly used terms in the passage and could be mistaken as relevant concepts. They are really just off-tangent concepts.

12. Correct Answer: C

This question requires recognising similarities between new information introduced and a significant concept discussed in the passage. The question specifies the ideas associated with the layman's term "romantic": love, affection, irrationality. These are then related to the concept that was developed by the Romantic Movement.

A and B are decoys that use outside knowledge and not discussed in the passage.

(C) This is discussed in the passage, particularly in P2 S3.

(D) This would sound highly relevant. However, this is only specific to Wordsworth's principle, not to Romanticism in general. Likewise, Wordsworth's claim does not address the concept of "irrationality".

13. Correct Answer: C

This question asks you to infer the qualities of an art genre that are not explicitly defined in the text. The passage defines Gauguin's work as a reaction against Impressionism, stating that "He wanted to portray the essence of things rather than the exterior form" and "not try to render the model exactly as one sees it". It also states that he reintroduced the outline to art. Thus the passage suggests that Impressionism was focussed on capturing reality exactly as it appeared to the eye. The correct choice is (C).

(A) The passage does not imply that Impressionist images were idealised, but that they were intended to represent things as they really appear.

(B) The passage emphasises representing an object "exactly as one sees it" and not as technical instruments show it to be.

(D) Although the passage does not explicitly exclude the use of bright and expressive colours and lines in Impressionist paintings, it clearly states that their subjects are literal representations of real objects and scenery. It is, therefore, safe to conclude that NO Impressionist painting is "a visual expression of emotional experiences".

14. Correct Answer: C

This question asks you to reason about possible similarities between two art movements that are described as opposites. The passage states that in Impressionism, one paints the work "exactly as one sees it" while in Symbolism, "painters try to give a visual expression to emotional experiences". Thus in both forms of painting, the artist tries to portray a subjective internal experience, whether sensory or emotional.

(A) This choice is incorrect because the passage never mentions ideas as a component of Impressionist works.

(B) The passage gives no reason to believe that all Symbolist paintings were based on observing nature.

(D) This choice is irrelevant because the passage never discusses the individual versus society.

15. Correct Answer: A

This question requires you to understand the author's main claims about Gauguin. The passage states that Gauguin's work "marked a break from the past" and describes him as a key originator of many aspects of Symbolism. If he instead borrowed these ideas and techniques from others, his influence and originality would be less, and his painting would represent less of a dramatic break from earlier work.

(B) This choice is irrelevant because the fact that both groups rejected an earlier style does not diminish the importance of the break between the two of them.

(C) This choice would reinforce the author's claims since the passage focusses on Gauguin's lack of interest in accuracy.

(D) This is also irrelevant because the passage does not imply that the Impressionists' work was never revolutionary.

16. Correct Answer: D

This question asks you to consider how quotes from artists relate to what we know about Gauguin's ideas. The quote from Manet suggests seeing the external world and capturing it immediately in a painting. This runs contrary to the ideas presented in the passage. The first paragraph says Gauguin was "preoccupied with suggestion rather than description" and that Symbolism is defined as the "rejection of direct, literal representation in favour of evocation and suggestion". This quote would thus align Manet with Impressionism, which Gauguin rejects.

(A) This quote from Cezanne presents another principle of simplification, which is consistent with the idea of the passage about Synthetism as well as Gauguin's reintroduction of "emphatic outlines".

(B) This quote is the exact antithesis of option (D) and suggests that painting should be based on expressing feeling, one of Symbolism's principles.

(C) This quote does not concern itself with the external world but the internal experience or soul of the artist.

17. Correct Answer: C

To answer this question, you have to look closely at what the passage says about Impressionism. The author never implies that Impressionist paintings were not beautiful.

(A) Paragraph 1 states that Gauguin abandoned Impressionism due to the limitations of the style.

(B) The passage states that Symbolists wanted paintings to "express the artists' emotions, sensibilities, and personal experiences of the world around them" (paragraph 4), suggesting that they would reject unemotional works.

(D) The Symbolists' "rejection of direct, literal representation" (paragraph 2) suggests they saw imagination as important.

18. Correct Answer: D

This question asks you to infer connections between Japanese painting and Gaugin's Synthetist-Symbolist art. Even without prior knowledge of Japanese art nor any discussions of it in the passage, the question itself implies that a reasonable assumption can be made using the descriptions provided in the passage about Synthetist-Symbolism.

Most of these descriptions are found in paragraph 4, particularly about how Gaugin used colours freely and "unnaturalistically for its decorative or emotional effect. . . the forms of his pictures were constructed from symbolic patterns of colour and linear rhythms". The correct answer is (D).

(A) The passage does state that Gauguin used outlines but does not suggest the importance of fluidity or curved versus straight lines.

(B) Paragraph 2 states that Symbolism, one of the two movements from which Gauguin formed his "new" art, has death, disease, and sin as its typical subjects. Gauguin similarly relates in paragraph 4 that "it was in himself that he searched rather than in his surroundings". This makes this answer choice incorrect.

(C) Gauguin was particularly interested in suggesting mental images and ideas in an art work as opposed to merely representing visual reality. Nothing in the passage mentions narrative as a factor in his artistic process or form.

19. Correct Answer: A

This type of question focusses on a general assessment of the passage as a whole and its main purpose. We must consider that all of the answers are partially correct, therefore the answer that is most inclusive will be correct. By doing this, we can assess that (A) encompasses all the others mentioned in (B), (C), and (D), as evidenced in the introductory sentence and Paragraph 7 in its entirety.

20. Correct Answer: C

This is a complex-sounding question, which requires a process of deduction. Again, we must look for the lateral distinction of inclusion to indicate the answer to this tone question. All the answers are partially correct, yet one will stand out from the others and include the other answers. There are passages which are (A) bleak, as well as (D) cautious, yet these are relatively too focussed to be general assessments of the "tone of the author." There are also indications of (B) some hope in the author's suggestions about wisdom and liberty, yet we cannot define the entire passage as "hopeful." (C) Existential is the most inclusive of the others because "existence will carry with it moments of caution, hope, as well as bleakness and despair." Despite its "absurdist" ring, the reflections of existential thought, found in Camus, Sartre, Ionesco, and others run the full range and gamut of human emotions and actions. The term existentialism has often been compared to a "tragic optimism" view of life, which this passage certainly suggests.

21. Correct Answer: D

This is a complex-sounding question and the answers are full of abstractions, which one must be very careful while ruling out answers.

(A) simply does not make sense – a created sort of joke and certainly does not go against the thesis.

(B) is a tangent and not really related to the author's thesis.

(C) is also a tangent and not really related to the author's thesis.

(D) would go against the author's "entropic" view of humankind. If this is considered to be true, even hypothetically, it would qualify as the best choice, given the other options.

22. Correct Answer: C

This detail-oriented question can be answered by a close reading particularly in Paragraph 7: We shall define philosophy as "total perspective," as mind overspreading life and forging chaos into unity.

23. **Correct Answer: D**
This is a best-option type of question, in which all of the answers may be partially correct or inferred and/or implicative of passage information. Only (D) answers the question directly and can be found in Paragraph 7:
Philosophy is harmonised knowledge making a harmonious life.

24. **Correct Answer: A**
This is a detail-oriented question based on a distinction which the author makes within the passage. The best ratio is (A) while the other answers are created distractions. This idea is reflected in the following statement, from the passage:
Knowledge is power, but only wisdom is liberty.
(B) A distraction – philosophical babble of existentialism
(C) Babble of philosophy in general
(D) Never mentioned

25. **Correct Answer: C**
This is an inference question based on modern affiliations of people with the internet.
(A) is too generalised. We cannot proclaim we all feel disconnected and shallow.
(B) is also too generalised; we cannot all proclaim we feel connected and hopeful.
(C) When on the internet, we feel interconnected yet disassociated. While this is a bit of a paradox because the context of face-to-face communication is not there, this is the best option.
(D) is too generalised, and the metaphor of a network is faulty. If there is a metaphor for the internet, the rhizome would be descriptive. Linear suggests one-way, we know that is untrue for the internet. There are multiple connections, going in multiple ways simultaneously constituting a quite complex assemblage of information and communication.

26. **Correct Answer: C**
Given the complexity of this question, which is based on detail and close reading or re-scan, one must be very careful because of the way terms are being emplaced together.
(A) This is too obvious and is somewhat tautological in reasoning (circular argument). If read carefully, it really does not answer the question.
(B) This is never really mentioned within the passage; this answer concerns linguistics.
(C) This is a summation of P2 S2 and answers the question.
(D) This is too obvious also and tautological, not really answering the question.

27. **Correct Answer: B**
This is an associative type of question where the answer must be the BEST choice or inference given the range of options:
(A) is partially true, yet "the abyss of chaos" is too extreme.
(B) This is the correct answer: the romantic imagery of the rose versus the destructive imagery of a worm flying through the storm making the rose sick.
(C) Linguistically, a real rose can be sick – infected with disease, bug-ridden, etc. This is an incorrect option.
(D) This answer is too general. Yes, there are multiple meanings and effects upon a reader, but that is a condition of most poetry.

28. **Correct Answer: D**
This question is another best-option type given the range of answers, in which one must deduce through a process of elimination (PoE) to arrive at the correct answer.
(A) Telescopic is vague and similar to (C), which is also incorrect. It suggests nothing of the author's attitude towards archetypes.
(B) Critical is also vague. This could be translated in a number of different ways – serious and analytical, which suggests more of an approach rather than an "attitude".
(C) This can be ruled out for a similar reason as

(A). (D) Archetypes as encompassing can be inferred to be correct because it is the theoretical framework of which the poem is analysed. Given the statements in P2, this idea can easily be supported.

29. Correct Answer: C

This is a detail-oriented question, which must be drawn from the passage itself because all of the answers may be implicative of the passage or inferred to be at least partially correct. Within the passage itself, (A) and (B) may be implied yet never directly mentioned as in (C) - Last Paragraph, S1. (D) is indicative of Blake yet overly complex and not mentioned within the passage.

30. Correct Answer: A

This type of question is also detail-oriented, which must be solved by close reading, rescan and deduction through the process of elimination (PoE).

(A) is implied in Paragraph 2.

(B) This answer is a created distraction – intention is never mentioned in the passage.

(C) and (D) are either too obvious or too literal to be correct yet lacks specificity.

31. Correct Answer: B

This type of question is also detail-oriented, which must be solved by close reading, rescan and deduction through the process of elimination (PoE).

(A) and (C) are tangential and unfocussed, therefore, incorrect. (D) is too specific yet likewise tangential and unfocussed. (B) can be affirmed by Paragraph 5 in general and thus correct.

32. Correct Answer: D

This complex-sounding question must proceed to be answered by the comparison of the poem with Milton:

(A) is partially true. The stories are the same, yet the language and style are quite different.

(B) is incorrect and a created tangent distraction amounting to nonsense, which means cannot be recovered(?).

(C) is also incorrect: the general theme of both poem and the Milton excerpt is quite similar.

(D) is correct. The similarities of the two almost border on weirdness given the general theme.

33. Correct Answer: C

Answering this question requires you to think about the author's tone. Crabb writes that critics of Godot "often turn red in the face fomenting on its inadequacies. It is mere gibberish, they cry, eyes nearly bulging out of their head". The passage aims to make these critics appear foolish by showing that their distaste for the play is exaggerated and overemotional. Thus his tone is mocking.

(A) This excerpt cannot be described as analytical since the language used is so emotionally weighted.

(B) The excerpt is based on describing a certain type of critic rather than persuading the reader of anything.

(D) This passage does not describe a concept or term.

34. Correct Answer: D

This question calls for an understanding of the passage's definition of a theatrical genre. According to a line quoted in the text, Absurd Theatre aims at "making man aware of the ultimate realities of his condition, by instilling in him again the lost sense of cosmic wonder and primaeval anguish. The Absurd Theatre hopes to achieve this by shocking man out of an existence that has become trite, mechanical and complacent." Thus this form of theatre intends to make viewers more aware of certain aspects of life, not just as they watch the play, but overall. The correct answer is (D).

I. The passage states that dialogue in *Waiting for Godot* is "ludicrous" and describes Theatre of the Absurd as opposed to realism.

II. While the passage does define these plays as possessing mythic elements, it also describes Waiting for Godot as an almost plotless play that "seems to end in precisely the same condition it began". This suggests absurdist plays can have plots quite unlike those of traditional mythic narratives.

35. Correct Answer: B

This question asks you to make inferences from the author's description of an unusual play. The passage states that characters "bide their time awaiting the arrival of Godot, but that in the end, nothing happens, describing its message as "Change...is only an illusion." Thus we can infer that the event the characters are waiting for does not happen and that this has implied significance for human life overall.

(A) We are told the characters "have difficulty communicating the simplest of concepts to one another." Thus they do not eloquently voice the author's views.

(C) The overall message of the play is described as invoking absurdity and futility, so its message is negative, not ambivalent.

(D) The passage describes the play's message as focussed on life overall, not on a specific time period or type of person.

36. Correct Answer: A

This question is asking you to understand the absurdist playwrights' described motivation. The passage states that they "attempt to convey their sense of bewilderment, anxiety, and wonder in the face of an inexplicable universe". It goes on to discuss "instilling in [man] again the lost sense of cosmic wonder and primaeval anguish". Thus the main purpose is to make life's absurdity palpable to viewers.

(B) The passage does suggest the plays shocked people, but not that this was their main purpose.

(C) The passage does not suggest that the plays are a "respite" but a disturbing experience that reflects life's troubling qualities.

(D) The passage suggests that the playwrights were attempting to convey an experience, but one that they consider a truth about life, not unique to their worldview.

37. Correct Answer: C

This question is asking what type of literary phenomenon Theatre of the Absurd is. A genre is a category of artistic production in which works are grouped together based on similarities in subject matter, style and form. The passage describes Theatre of the Absurd as a type of play whose authors shared similar thematic concerns and means (such as static plots) of achieving them. This fits the definition of a genre.

(A) The passage describes Theatre of the Absurd as distinct from realism and rejecting the need to portray reality accurately.

(B) The passage never states Theatre of the Absurd had widespread influence on later forms of theatre.

(D) A template suggests a rigid set of instructions that would result in similar works while the passage describes a more loose set of interests and theatrical devices.

38. Correct Answer: C

In this question, candidates must be able to understand the author's overall concept of woman as the "Other". The passage describes man as one who "will provide woman-the-liege with material protection and will undertake the moral justification of her existence" implying that it is the man who takes the significant role of the provider while the woman settles for the convenience of being his dependent. This makes option (C) correct.

(A) This is a close answer because the author refers to the woman as a "liege" (which could either mean a slave or a dependent) who feels a "necessary bond that ties her to man". However, this is only because the woman's option of individuality is difficult that she chooses this role of subordination as indicated by the line: "But it is an easy road; on it, one avoids the strain involved in undertaking an authentic existence." In other words, a woman is not entirely a slave who is bound to obey without any choice but more of a willing dependent.

(B) A communal partnership is also close in the sense that the nature of this type of relationship is based on providing benefits and looking out for the welfare of the other person. However, the role of each person in the relationship is that of a partner - not as a sovereign to his subordinate as the passage author describes.

(D) Nothing is mentioned about conspiracy in the passage.

39. Correct Answer: C

The beginning of the paragraph places emphasis on change in the world as women are "beginning to take part in the affairs of the world" but makes reference to the pre-existing state of the world where it "belongs to men". This distinction between the status quo and the changes that are starting to occur in women's place in the world emphasises the existence of "social preconditions" that dictate the unequal roles of men and women. (A) and (D) are some of the reasons implied in the passage why women submit to their subordinate role in society. The author describing society as (B) male-oriented only reinforces the fact that the importance accorded to the role of men is socially preconditioned.

40. Correct Answer: B

This question requires differentiating the author's concept of women as the (A) dependent "Other" from what she explains to be women's self-perception as (B) willing subordinates of men. The last line of the passage details the circumstances that lead women to conveniently acquiesce to their subordinate role in a male-oriented society. This question is asking candidates to determine how a woman considers herself based on passage information, and this is best answered by option (B). Answer choice (C) would require a subjective interpretation of the passage, which is incorrect. The passage briefly states that men "undertake the moral justification of [women's] existence" but this does not necessarily imply that women perceive themselves as (D) man's moral responsibility.

High-level Importance

SPOILER ALERT

Gold Standard has cross-referenced the content in this chapter to examples from ACER's official GAMSAT practice materials. It is for you to decide when you want to explore these questions since you may want to preserve some of ACER's materials for timed mock-exam practice.

Examples – Sociology Q30-35 and 65-72 of 3, Q1-6, Q27-31 and Q37-41 of 4, Q35-40 of 5; Literature and Arts Q1-8 of 1, Q66-72 of 4; Philosophy Q13-21 of 2, Q13-17 and Q56-60 of 3; History and Culture - Q1-10, Q13-21 of 1, Q15-20 and Q21-24 of 5. Note that "Q" is followed by the question number, and, for example, "of 1" refers to booklet number 1 which is referenced in the Spoiler Alert table at the end of section RHSS 3.2.4. The 15 full-length HEAPS GAMSAT practice tests (by Gold Standard) include exams that contain specific cross-references to this chapter within the worked solutions.

Chapter Checklist

- ☐ Access your online account to view answers, worked solutions and discussion boards.
- ☐ Complete a maximum of 1 page of notes using symbols/abbreviations to represent the content in the foregoing section. These are your Gold Notes.
- ☐ Consider your options based on your optimal way of learning:
    - ☐ Create your own, tangible study cards or try the free app: Anki.
    - ☐ Record your voice reading your Gold Notes onto your smartphone (MP3s) and listen during exercise, transportation, etc.
    - ☐ Consider reading at least 1 source material every day (e.g., poems of a single author, a synopsis of a novel, an article from a scientific journal that caught your interest, etc.). Note down the main idea or ideas of the piece on your scratch paper. Determine or surmise the author's sentiment or purpose for writing the material.
- ☐ Reassess your schedule for your full-length GAMSAT practice tests: ACER and/or HEAPS exams. Ensure that you have scheduled one full day to complete a practice test and 1-2 days for a thorough assessment of worked solutions while adding to your abbreviated Gold Notes.
- ☐ Reassess your progress in scheduling and/or evaluating stress reduction techniques such as regular exercise (sports), yoga, meditation and/or mindfulness exercises (*see* YouTube for suggestions).

3.8.3 Verbal Reasoning Exercise 2 (Science-based Passages)

The following is a sample mini test which is designed to aid in developing your skills in reading and answering passages that are related to science or medicine. These types of passages are known to appear in Reasoning in Humanities and Social Sciences of recent GAMSATs.

There are 7 Units with 40 questions. Choose the best answer for each question. You have 60 minutes. Please time yourself.

BEGIN ONLY WHEN TIMER IS READY.

Unit 1

Questions 1 - 5

Gold was first discovered at Summitville mine in Colorado in 1870. Significant gold production from underground workings occurred prior to 1900. In 1903, the Reynolds adit (entrance for access, drainage, and ventilation) was driven to drain the underground workings and serve as an ore haulage tunnel. Production occurred sporadically through the 1950s. The district received some exploration attention in the 1970s as a copper prospect, but no mining for copper was pursued.

Similar to many historic gold mining districts in the western United States, Summitville received renewed interest in the early 1980s due to technological advances that allow extraction of low-grade ores with cyanide heap leach techniques. In 1984, Summitville Consolidated Mining Company, Inc. (SCMCI), initiated open pit mining of gold ore from rocks surrounding the historic underground workings, where gold concentrations had been too low to be economic for the underground mining operations. Ore from the pit was crushed and placed on a heap leach pad overlying a protective liner. Cyanide solutions were sprinkled onto the heap and trickled down through the crushed ore, dissolving the gold. The processing solutions were then collected from the base of the heap leach pile, and the gold was chemically extracted from the solutions.

Environmental problems developed soon after the initiation of open-pit mining. Acidic, metal rich drainage into the Wightman Fork of the Alamosa River increased significantly from numerous sources on site, including the Reynolds adit and the Cropsy waste dump. Cyanide-bearing processing solutions began leaking into an underdrain system beneath the heap leach pad, where they then mixed with acid ground waters from the Cropsy waste dump. Cyanide solutions also leaked from transfer pipes directly into the Wightman Fork several times over the course of mining.

SCMCI had ceased active mining and had begun environmental remediation when it declared bankruptcy in December 1992 and abandoned the mine site. The bankruptcy created several immediate concerns. Earlier in 1992, the company had brought a water treatment plant on line to begin treating the estimated 150 to 200 million gallons of spent cyanide processing solutions remaining in the heap; however, treatment was proceeding so slowly relative to influx of snowmelt waters that the waters were in danger of overtopping a containment dike and flowing directly into the Wightman Fork. In addition, piping carrying the processing solutions to the treatment plant would have frozen within several hours, releasing cyanide solutions and stopping water treatment.

At the request of the State of Colorado, the U.S. Environmental Protection Agency (EPA) immediately took over the site under EPA Superfund Emergency Response authority and increased treatment of the heap leach solutions, thereby averting a catastrophic release of cyanide solutions from the heap. Summitville was added to the EPA National Priorities List in late May 1994. Ongoing remediation efforts include decommissioning of the heap leach pad, plugging of the Reynolds and Chandler adits, backfilling of the open pit with acid-generating mine waste material, and capping of the backfilled pit to prevent water inflow. The total cost of the cleanup has been estimated to be from US $100 million to $120 million.

The environmental problems at Summitville have been of particular concern due to the extensive downstream use of Alamosa River water for livestock, agricultural irrigation, and wildlife habitat. Increased acid and metal loadings from Summitville are suspected to have caused the 1990 disappearance of stocked fish from Terrace Reservoir and farm holding ponds along the Alamosa River. The Alamosa River is used extensively to irrigate crops in the southwestern San Luis Valley. Important crops include alfalfa (used for livestock feed), barley (used in beer production), wheat, and potatoes; there has been concern about potential adverse effects of the increased acid and metal loadings from Summitville on the metal content and viability of these crops. The Alamosa River also feeds wetlands that are habitat for aquatic life and migratory water fowl such as ducks and the endangered whooping crane; there are concerns about Summitville's effects on these wetlands and their associated wildlife.

- U.S. Department of the Interior | U.S. Geological Survey

1. What is the main idea of the passage?

A. Open pit mining has disastrous effects.
B. Open pit mining in Summitville has caused pending environmental hazards.
C. There is a need for stricter controls and regulations governing open pit mining.
D. Open pit mining typically affects the environment.

2. What is the author's purpose of the passage?

A. To demonstrate and warn of the potential harmful effects left by Summitville mining to the environment, particularly the Alamosa River
B. To illustrate the environmental need for legislation for all open pit mining areas
C. To demonstrate and suggest that similar efforts in other areas should follow the Summitville mining "cleanup" protocol and agenda
D. To rally support for environmental groups and their political eco-green proposals and agenda

3. What evidence would **most strongly** support the author's argument?

A. Cyanide toxins can contaminate wetlands downstream in typical mining areas.
B. The disappearance of certain species has been noted due to open pit mining.
C. There are neither regulatory controls in place for the monitoring of toxins nor clean-up planning in case of emergencies.
D. Open pit mining threatens all life in as much as it threatens the general ecosystem of the area.

4. According to passage information, which of the following were **not** potentially affected by the runoff into the Alamosa River?

I. Wildlife habitat
II. Potable drinking water
III. Livestock

A. I and III
B. II only
C. III only
D. II and III

5. What are the dominant kinds of evidence or support used by the author to strengthen his or her thesis?

A. Real examples and statistics
B. Hypothetical examples and statistics
C. Expert testimony and current regulations
D. Emotional appeals and green reasoning

Unit 2

Questions 6 - 11

Alfred Adler was a Viennese physician who founded Adlerian Psychology. He was the first in the fields of psychiatry and psychology to stress the importance of our perceptions and social relationships in affecting our emotional and physical health, as well as the health of our families and communities. The following passage discusses the main principles of Adlerian Psychology.

Adlerian Psychology holds that human beings are goal-oriented and choice-making by nature, not mechanistically victims of instinct, drives, and environment. As social beings, our basic goal is to belong. Although heredity and environment have strong influences, to a large extent, we make our own choices of how to belong.

Adlerian Psychology has a strong focus on prevention of mental disturbance and social distress through education and parenting. Much of Adler's work was with teachers and parents who wanted to replace traditional authoritarian styles of relating to children with more democratic—but not permissive—ways. One of Adlerian Psychology's claims to fame is the attribution to Adlerian Psychology of the concept that "separate is not equal" by an author of the social science brief for the US Supreme Court case on school desegregation. Today, many schools incorporate Adlerian-based approaches in teacher training and classroom work, and many parenting courses throughout the country are Adlerian-based.

Adler's concept of *Gemeinschaftsgefühl*, or a deep sense of fellowship in the human community and interconnectedness with all life, holds that human beings, as social beings, have a natural desire to contribute usefully for the good of humanity. According to Adler, a desire for social significance must focus on contribution, not on status-seeking, or one's social relationships and one's mental health will suffer.

Adlerian psychology is perhaps best known for the concept of the inferiority complex. Adler viewed some behaviour as overcompensation for perceived shortcomings. We sometimes make choices about how to belong on the basis of an often mistaken feeling of inferiority. Children, for example, sometimes seem to believe, mistakenly and not consciously, that they belong only when they are the centre of attention. Some adults act as if they believe, mistakenly, that they belong only when they can control others, or take revenge on others, or withdraw from others (and often such misperceptions developed in early childhood).

Both the inferiority complex and overcompensation indicated to Adler an exaggerated concern with self. This self-concern could be eased by nurturing one's innate abilities to cooperate and contribute through what Adler called the life tasks: work, intimacy, and friendship. Adlerian therapy helps to "liberate" clients by helping them move toward a clearer understanding of their unconscious, inferiority-based belief systems, or "lifestyles" and toward a clearer understanding of ways to incorporate cooperation and contribution and mutual respect in their relationships. Adlerians hope to let go of "private logic" and embrace dignity and respect in all relationships, thereby becoming emotionally and physically healthier and creating a more democratic culture.

- Adapted from Adlerian Psychology: An Overview (www.psasadler.org)

6. According to the passage, people's most important motive when interacting with others is to:

A. make choices.
B. perform tasks effectively.
C. be accepted.
D. overcome overcompensation.

7. Which of the following behaviours best exemplifies Adler's concept of *Gemeinschaftsgefühl?*

A. A person going on a hunger strike in response to social injustice
B. Running for political office to advance one's most important beliefs
C. A teacher giving a lecture on social justice history to her students
D. Ecological involvement with a local green group

8. It can be assumed from passage information that Adler's philosophies were in conflict with all of the following **except** those of:

A. Skinner, who argued that behaviour is determined by its consequence and will be repeated if it is positively reinforced.
B. Freud, who argued that behaviour is shaped by drives and psychological features like the Oedipus complex.
C. Maslow, who postulated that people have a hierarchy of needs ranging from basic survival to esteem and self-actualisation.
D. Ayn Rand, who argued that people should consider their perceptions and logic the only true authority and their happiness the ultimate moral goal.

9. Based on passage information, one can ascertain that a person's mental health in Adlerian Psychology is primarily based on:

- **A.** overcompensation and inferiority complexes.
- **B.** innate abilities and the ability to achieve goals.
- **C.** fulfilment of instinctual desires.
- **D.** social outlook and interaction.

10. Based on passage information, what is typical of behaviour based on an inferiority complex?

- **A.** It displays an outsize need to impress others.
- **B.** It is self-deprecating and overly modest.
- **C.** It is designed to avoid attracting attention.
- **D.** It reveals the subject's paradoxical desire to prove their inferiority.

11. We might infer that according to Adler, ways to improve psychological health would include all of the following **except**:

- **A.** undergoing psychotherapy to find out what false assumptions one is holding onto.
- **B.** undergoing testing to learn one's personality type to find a suitable job.
- **C.** practising productive ways to react when feelings of inferiority surface.
- **D.** finding ways to treat friends and loved ones with more respect.

Unit 3

Questions 12 - 16

In the natural sciences, enquiry is concerned with uncovering or discovering that which exists. "Invention" is not considered to be a feature of scientific enquiry and is perhaps not compatible with the dispassionate relationship with knowledge that scientists have traditionally claimed. Design, by contrast, claims invention (and personal ownership of it) as a central principle so it is difficult at first to see where the two traditions can overlap.

A central problem of science is how to recognise and define worthwhile subjects for investigation. For one thing, we may be faced with a myriad of opportunities and no means to decide which are going to be fruitful. On the other hand, our environment may limit our ability to recognise scientific problems and possibilities, especially the ones which could lead to significant changes in our understanding. To illustrate this second problem, philosophers have speculated on the science and culture of imaginary worlds which have fundamentally different and more restricted conditions than ours. If you and your environment consist of gases with no solid objects to reflect on, then you may not be able to conceive of geometry as we know it. If you lived in a 1- or 2-dimensional world you would have a very different set of concepts from us and, no doubt, people living in a 5-dimensional world would see us as conceptually impoverished in much the same way. Artists also engage with these issues, often in stimulating and accessible forms. For example, science fiction writers explore imaginary worlds which shape their civilisations in ways that may inform us about our own experience. Brian Aldiss described a world where each season lasted for many lifetimes, including a harsh winter which few people and institutions survived, effectively cutting people off from their history and most of the knowledge acquired during the previous summer. This fictional device provided a fresh perspective for the examination of individuals and societies confronted with difficult circumstances.

These abstracted questions have their parallels in everyday life and more mundane enquiries. Michael Polanyi describes the 'logical gap' between existing knowledge and any significant discovery or innovation. No matter how thorough our factual knowledge of the situation that we inhabit, the pursuit of logical reasoning or iterative development of existing concepts would not, on its own, allow us to cross this gap. There must be also some kind of leap of 'illumination' by which the scientist imagines a new concept and proposes it as a worthwhile subject for investigation. As Polanyi says, "Illumination....is the plunge by which we gain a foothold in another shore of reality. On such plunges, the scientist has to stake, bit by bit, his entire professional life."

Polanyi was concerned with what he called the "tacit dimension" in our knowledge. In particular, he wished to give proper value to the process of recognising, and making a commitment to, ideas or hypotheses, which may result from a rich understanding and knowledge but cannot be explained by explicit reasoning, in order to carry out the enquiry that will lead to them being more widely understood and accepted. I have used the term "accepted" rather than "proved" (itself shorthand for Karl Popper's concept of a falsifiable hypothesis that has proved so far to be reliable) because Polanyi held that all scientific knowledge is a question of "passionate belief" rather than dispassionate proof, requiring us to take account of the methods, competence, judgement and integrity of scientists, and the knowledge and principles that we already hold, before we accept the knowledge which they offer us. This seems much more reasonable today when more people appreciate the limitations of science than 50 years ago when Polanyi was developing his ideas.

High-level Importance

12. The crux of the problem, which the author specifically focusses on is:
- **A.** developing protocol for what scientific endeavours are advisable to pursue.
- **B.** how scientific invention is related to discovery.
- **C.** the idea that scientific knowledge is a question of passionate belief.
- **D.** the idea that scientific knowledge is a question of dispassionate proof.

13. The relevance or significance of the passage, in relation to scientific invention and discovery, concerns:
- **A.** knowledge.
- **B.** criteria.
- **C.** instrumentation.
- **D.** measurement.

14. According to passage information, Polyani makes a distinction between tacit knowledge and what can be inferred as knowledge which is:
- **A.** socially constructed.
- **B.** hypothetically determined.
- **C.** explicit reasoning.
- **D.** deductively reasoned.

15. According to passage information, for Polyani, "illumination" is:
- **I.** the key to invention and discovery in scientific endeavour.
- **II.** the bridge over the logical gap between theory and application.
- **III.** the connection between innovation and what is already known.

- **A.** I only
- **B.** II only
- **C.** II and III
- **D.** I and III

16. The author pursues the notion of which central problem that may limit our ability to recognise scientific problems and possibilities?
- **A.** Instrumentation designed to measure phenomena
- **B.** Knowledgeable processes involved in research
- **C.** Methodologies which are employed in measurement
- **D.** Environment or setting surrounding us

Unit 4

Questions 17 - 23

The politicisation of science is the manipulation of science for political gain. It occurs when government, business, or advocacy groups use legal or economic pressure to influence the findings of scientific research or the way it is disseminated, reported or interpreted. The politicisation of science may also negatively affect academic and scientific freedom. Historically, groups have conducted various campaigns to promote their interests in defiance of scientific consensus, and in an effort to manipulate public policy.

In August 2003, United States Democratic Congressman Henry A. Waxman and the staff of the Government Reform Committee released a report concluding that the administration of George W. Bush had politicised science and sex education. The report accuses the administration of modifying performance measures for abstinence-based programmes to make them look more effective. The report also found that the Bush administration had appointed Dr. Joseph McIlhaney, a prominent advocate of abstinence-only programme, to the Advisory Committee to the director of the Centre for Disease Control. According to the report, information about comprehensive sex education was removed from the CDC's website.

The Union of Concerned Scientists (UCS) also issued a report indicating that the Bush administration delayed for nine months an EPA report (eventually leaked) that indicated that 8 percent of women between the ages of 16 and 49 have blood mercury levels that could lead to reduced I.Q. and motor skills in their offspring. When new rules of mercury emissions were finally released by the EPA, at least 12 paragraphs were transferred, sometimes verbatim, from a legal document prepared by industry attorneys.

According to the Waxman Report, other issues considered for removal from government sponsored programmes included agricultural pollution, the Arctic National Wildlife Refuge and breast cancer; the report found that a National Cancer Institute website has been changed to reflect the administration view that there may be a risk of breast cancer associated with abortions. The website was updated after protests and now holds that no such risk has been found in recent, well-designed studies. In addition, proponents of "Intelligent Design" (ID) over "Evolution" have government-spearheaded efforts to be entered into the public schools and with success.

The overwhelming majority of the scientific community, which supports theories that are testable by experiment or observation, oppose treating ID, which is neither a scientific theory.

High-level Importance

A 1999 report by the National Academy of Sciences states, “Creationism, intelligent design, and other claims of supernatural intervention in the origin of life or of species are not science because they are not testable by the methods of science.” Public officials have supported public schools teaching intelligent design alongside evolution in science curricula.

In January 2007, the House Committee on Science and Technology announced the formation of a new subcommittee, the Science Subcommittee on Investigations and Oversight, which handles investigative and oversight activities on matters covering the committee's entire jurisdiction. The subcommittee has the authority to look into a whole range of important issues, particularly those concerning manipulation of scientific data at Federal agencies.

In an interview, subcommittee chairman Rep. Brad Miller pledged to "look into. . . scientific integrity issues under the Bush Administration. There have been lots of reports in the press of manipulating science to support policy, rigging advisory panels, and suppressing research by federal employees or with federal dollars. I've written about that here before, and you interviewed me a year ago about the manipulation of science. In addition to the published reports, the committee staff has been collecting accounts, some confidential, of interference by political appointees.” Yet the promised reports were far from adequate (two educational reports) or not released completely to the public, quite possibly due to bipartisan politics and mutual scratch-back negotiations concerning other political agendas.

The issue is far from over. Patrick Michaels, as recently as April 2011, had written (CATO Institute), covering the climate change controversy, that "The conflation of political agendas with science is destroying the credibility of academia, with the complicity of the editors of our major scientific journals," noting a recent SCIENCE article which attempted to revive a 19th Century idea of "climatic determinism" - people do good things when things get warmer, bad things when cold – obviously, politically motivated.

17. What is the author’s main argument in this passage?

- **A.** The Bush administration has been the worst offender in politicising science.
- **B.** Politicisation of science is common and a serious danger to evidence-based public policy.
- **C.** Accurate scientific information usually supports liberal policies, not conservative.
- **D.** It can be difficult to tell when a scientific claim by a politician or government agency is truthful.

18. "Abstinence-based programmes" (paragraph 2) refer to:
- **A.** information campaigns advocated by the people.
- **B.** ideological assumptions that promote reproductive choices.
- **C.** democratic agendas on preventing teen pregnancy.
- **D.** comprehensive sex education information campaigns.

19. Which of the following would count as a politicisation of science?
- **A.** Cherry-picking studies that suggest US nutrition guidelines are healthy and citing only those studies in a press release
- **B.** Using data from a new climate study to push for stricter environmental regulation
- **C.** Telling the public Iraq had weapons of mass destruction when it did not
- **D.** Conducting a study on the effects of welfare in an attempt to prove that more robust welfare programs benefit families

20. What of the following would the author likely **not** support to prevent the politicisation of science?
- **A.** Neutral oversight boards scrutinising the scientific claims of government agencies and political parties
- **B.** Less emphasis on science as a basis for political decisions
- **C.** Decisions about what to include in science curricula being based on the consensus among practising scientists
- **D.** New regulations that do not allow scientific reports from government agencies to be delayed or withheld from the public

21. The quoted statement by Rep. Brad Miller in paragraph 7 suggests that the passage author thinks it was:
- **A.** mendacious.
- **B.** unreliable.
- **C.** falsely-advertised.
- **D.** politically-motivated.

22. Which of the following does the author **not** state is a problem with intelligent design?
- **A.** The people promoting it have a political agenda.
- **B.** It cannot be proven true or false through scientific experiment.
- **C.** It is not supported as a valid theory by practising scientists.
- **D.** It is controversial and offends many people.

23. What does the passage imply to be a likely reason that reports by the Science Subcommittee on Investigations and Oversight were not fully released to the public?

A. Politicians conspired to suppress reports containing information that was not flattering to anyone.

B. No one understood the importance of the reports, so they were ignored.

C. Democrats had little power during that time period and could not force Republicans to release them.

D. Selected reports were concealed in exchange for political favours.

Unit 5

Questions 24 - 28

It has become more and more common to link together the once disparate concepts of biology and morality. One such way of doing this, which some sociobiologists have advocated, is by introducing the idea of "epigenetic rules". Epigenetic rules mean something like the following: there are certain genetically based processes that are realised in chemically and structurally similar ways in all (or most) humans. For example, there are specific patterns of neurotransmitters and organisational features of fibres and brain tissue that develop in more or less the same fashion in all humans, and this development is somehow regulated, though not determined, by our genes. By influencing and shaping the physical and consequently cognitive processes of the brain, genes affect, but do not determine, the range of possibilities humans possess. Epigenetic rules, then, are the sorts of processes that both constrain and predispose humans to behave and think within a certain range of options. Often cited as examples are certain phobias that transcend cultural boundaries; people tend to fear the dark, high places, snakes, etc.

These epigenetic constraints and dispositions are not limited to simple behaviours and perceptions, but also to our moral sense; epigenetic rules provide a boundary for what humans consider moral. For example, epigenetic rules may predispose us to consider altruism a virtue, since there is an evolutionary advantage (or so some geneticists claim) for altruism; from a genetic point of view, altruistic acts often involve sacrificing the genes of one organism for the furthering of the gene pool of the entire population.

While this is unquestionably a provocative perspective, there are many points with which to take issue. It first seems that this thesis runs the risk of claiming that any common behaviour that transcends cultures and time periods may now be easily attributable to epigenetic rules. As one opponent of this view proposed, there are certain truths about humans, such as 'all humans have a tendency to throw spears pointy-end first'. This behaviour is observed in most cultures ('spears' can be replaced with 'pointy-edged object'), yet it is not at all clear that such behaviour is evidence that humans are genetically predisposed toward this. Rather, it seems that given a certain amount of intelligence and interaction with our environment, many different cultures will reach similar conclusions about which end of a spear proves the most effective. At the least, it is a very open question why humans exhibit similar behaviour patterns. In some cases our intuitions side more with genetics, in others, such as the example above, it seems that other factors are at work.

Further, merely knowing that a particular moral inclination has a genetic basis does not indicate how wrong it is to kill innocent people, so even if it could be shown that this sentiment has a genetic basis, it is possible to override or at least temper it. To put it more generally, just because morality has a basis in our genes (if it in fact does), it does not follow that we should look to our genes to generate, or even help out with, a theory of morality. As the philosopher Friedrich Nietzsche pointed out, explaining the origin of something like morality does not explain why it is successful, nor does the origin necessarily hold the key to explaining or furthering or even affecting its success.

24. The central point of the passage is that:
- **A.** epigenetic rules exist, it is just a matter of carefully researching their content.
- **B.** epigenetic rules may exist, but sociobiologists have been too hasty in claiming that they do.
- **C.** epigenetic rules probably exist, but sociobiologists should focus on different behaviours to determine the content of the rules.
- **D.** epigenetic rules do not exist.

25. The author's statement, "epigenetic rules may predispose us to consider altruism a virtue, since there is an evolutionary advantage to altruism" (paragraph 2) assumes that:
- **A.** epigenetic rules favour evolutionary advantages.
- **B.** epigenetic rules are themselves evolutionary advantages.
- **C.** altruism is an evolutionary advantage.
- **D.** what was considered an evolutionary advantage in the past may not be considered to be one currently.

High-level Importance

26. Based on the information in the last paragraph, the author would most likely agree with which of the following statements?

A. The fields of science and morality should remain separate.
B. The fact that most humans do not condone killing innocent people indicates the existence of epigenetic rules.
C. Genetic discoveries should not be strongly relied on to provide solutions to moral dilemmas.
D. Until research has unquestionably proven that there are relevant connections, we should not look to science to provide answers to moral dilemmas.

27. Which of the following is a claim made by the author but **not** supported in the passage by evidence, explanation, or example?

A. Epigenetic rules transcend cultural and historical boundaries.
B. Epigenetic rules influence conceptions of morality.
C. Not all similarities between humans have a genetic basis.
D. Explaining the origin of something does not explain why it is successful.

28. A recent study suggests that people living in rural areas fear snakes much more than gunshots while people living in urban areas fear gunshots more than snakes. These findings:

A. support the author's views.
B. support the sociobiologists' views.
C. indicate that neither is correct.
D. indicate that both are correct.

Unit 6

Questions 29 - 34

An "ethics of science" refers to ethical problems involved with scientific research, discoveries, and inventions. In scientific research and invention, experiments on humans, invention of biological weapons, etc., are scientific issues that assume ethical importance. In the field of medicine, ethical problems are associated with issues such as medical research, genetic manipulation, abortion, and euthanasia. In the field of environmental concerns, environmental ethics assumes an important place, as well.

The general issues that give rise to ethical questions concern scientific research and invention. In 1964, an experiment was carried out by the American psychologist Stanley Milgram that involved fooling people into thinking they were inflicting increasingly severe electric shocks on unseen but protesting victims. This experiment raised the ethical issue of whether it was morally right for a scientist to encourage people to inflict pain on others for experimental purposes. The issue of the invention of biological weapons that could affect civilians is an ethical one in the sense that it concerns the rightness or wrongness of harming civilians in war. The whole issue revolves around the concept of crime against humanity. One other issue related also to medicine is the issue of cloning, in which humans prescribe the genes of clones. How would a cloned child see his individuality after knowing that he was a clone? Wouldn't he feel his individuality as forever compromised? What if things go awry in the cloning process? Would that constitute a crime against a human? Who would be held responsible if things go awry?

Medical ethics is the study of moral standards in relation to the field of medicine. The ultimate issues underlying medical ethics are issues such as the definition of life and the value of life that are seen in the perspective of ethical theories regarding what differentiates good acts and principles from evil. Two of the problems, viz., medical research and embryo research will be discussed here. Research in medicine has the objective of alleviating human pain. However, this requires a study of how the human body works and what new drugs could be safely used to alleviate human pain. Things like experiments with embryos and test of drugs on humans assume ethical character when considering issues such as the value of life and the moral aim of medicine. For instance, during the 1980s there was a widespread debate about the ethics of research using human embryos. In such research, the embryos used were destroyed after 14 days from fertilisation. The argument that ended the debate in the UK leading to the legitimising of such research, up to the 14-day limit, was that a pre-14-day embryo was not in a state to be treated as an individual person since its cells were not differentiated to fulfil specific functions along with the possibility that the embryo was still in a condition to split into two identical twins. The 14-day limit assumed that since the nervous system begins to develop at about the 15th day from fertilisation, there was nothing ethically wrong with destroying it on the 14th day since the embryo doesn't know that it is a person. This also justifies abortion before the 14th day and provides a kind of ethical basis for research in human cloning.

The several assumptions behind the legalising of embryo research are that ethics is related to persons and not to potential persons, that personality is a matter of the nervous system and not the organism housing such a system, that humans are not accountable to anyone other than humans for what they do with any phenomenon of life; in other words, since God or some absolute judicial system doesn't exist, humans can decide what is to be done with humans. Such assumptions, however, cannot be accepted as axiomatic; they are philosophical issues, of course, but also crucial as pertaining to human life itself. In their ultimate development, such issues are settled according to the religious or anti-religious mindset of the political or judicial system in which the issues are raised.

29. According to the author, what was considered unethical about the Milgram experiment?

A. Some of the subjects suffered physically because they suffered from electric shocks.

B. The experimenters encouraged the subjects to behave cruelly by inflicting what they believed were electric shocks.

C. Some of the subjects suffered fear because they believed they were going to be shocked.

D. The experimenters were dishonest because they told the subjects beforehand that the electrical shocks were not real.

30. What would constitute a possible argument **against** anti-cloning arguments?

A. The process is so fascinating on a scientific level that the pros outweigh the cons.

B. Only a small number of people would have to be cloned to evaluate its effect on them.

C. Twins and triplets have duplicate DNA, yet they do not suffer identity crises.

D. Cloning is no different from other ways of scientifically creating life such as test tube babies.

31. What is the main idea of the passage?

A. An ethics of science concerns different disciplines and fields.

B. Scientific ethics, particularly in the medical field, are marked by controversy.

C. The ethics of science is a philosophical, not scientific, issue.

D. Ethical questions basically concern research and invention.

32. What is a possible rationale for experimenting on embryos only before the 14-day limit?

A. Because they cannot feel pain, they cannot be harmed.

B. Because they do not have specific human organs, they are potential rather than actual humans.

C. Because they do not have a personality and free will, they have no legitimate interest in life.

D. Because they are not yet viable outside the womb, they are not autonomous human beings.

33. What does the term "axiomatic" (last paragraph) mean?

A. Biased
B. Redundant
C. Needing further elaboration
D. Taken for granted

34. In the second paragraph, the author uses rhetorical questions to emphasise cloning's ethical issues. How does this **best** function in terms of providing evidence?

A. It lets the reader know that the questions are essentially unsolved.
B. The questions propel the reader to contemplate certain issues and think about how ethical questions affect them.
C. It stimulates the reader's emotions by showing that scientists are often shockingly unethical.
D. The examples given have similar solutions suggesting that the author's preferred ethical philosophy is correct.

Unit 7

Questions 35 - 40

Some would argue that with capitalism came the notion that society is best understood as the autonomous actions of individuals. This idea has its biological correlate in Darwin's theory of natural selection where evolution takes place at the level of the reproduction of individuals in a species. In science, in general, we find it in the reductionist assumption that the whole is best understood in terms of its parts, and the more minute the level one goes to, the better the explanation.

This way of conceptualising the world also has the effect of breaking up the world into autonomous domains: internal and external. Views of causation are also affected in that causes become referred to as either internal or external. Internal factors (genes) cause organisms to be the way they are and the external environment causes some organisms to be selected for and thereby to survive into the next generation.

One might assert that this is the way in which biology has been conceived since Darwin, and that it is a terribly impoverished way of viewing biology, and that our understanding of nature would be richer if we moved away from our reductionist tendencies and instead recognised the complex interaction of the organism with the environment it creates. We would also be more effective in solving our problems if we moved away from the tendency to focus merely on the proximal physiological causes of disease, for example, focusing on the bacteria or viruses associated with disease instead of social factors.

These proposals to avoid pure reductionism and to take into account causes other than physiological ones are well founded. But by implying that the traditional focus on physiological causes is merely an intricate way of masking the social cause behind the disease, one ignores the more innocuous motivations for picking physiological causes before social ones.

First, it must be said that no legitimate medical scientist or physician would claim that there is merely one cause - the cause - for nearly any disease. When it is said in science textbooks that something is the cause of something else what is really being said is something is the proximal physiological cause of something else. It is proximal because it is the nearer to the effect (disease process) and physiological because it itself is some biological or chemical agent (i.e. not a social agent). People may be troubled by western medicine's overemphasis of these causes as opposed to social ones. However, there seem to be very good, socially unproblematic reasons for often choosing to put the emphasis on the proximal physiological causes of disease.

Second, there is a logical reason. Consider bacteria and viruses. Wherever there is tuberculosis there is tubercle bacillus bacteria. The bacteria are a necessary condition for someone having the disease. The same cannot be said of sweat shops or unregulated, industrialised capitalism. In fact, individuals in the upper class and rural areas, as well as individuals in nonindustrial Marxist countries have also become infected by tubercle bacillus bacteria and come down with tuberculosis. This is not to say that for something to be labelled a cause of disease it must be a necessary condition, but the logical relationship of necessity helps us understand the claim that something is the cause of something else.

In addition, giving a necessary condition of disease does not limit one to saying that the cause of disease must be a proximal physiological one. Chewing tobacco releases toxic chemicals, which may be the cause of a specific form of gum disease in the chewer. Wherever this form of gum disease is found so is a user of chewing tobacco. In this case, it would seem perfectly appropriate to say that chewing tobacco is a cause of the disease, although not the proximal physiological one.

Finally, a reformed orientation toward science and medicine will yield a more fruitful way of doing investigations. Short-sighted causal explanation allows for the social structure to go unexamined for its deleterious effects on the community, but physiological explanations are important in determining the cause and potential solutions, both physiological and social.

35. What does the author mean by "capitalism . . . has its biological correlate in Darwin's theory of evolution"?

A. Both focus on complex relationships between groups of organisms and their surroundings.

B. Both are of the opinion that the more detailed level one goes to, the better the explanation.

C. Both hold a 'survival of the fittest' framework, e.g., the most successful organism will survive and reproduce.

D. Both hold the view that explanations are most effective when looking at individual entities.

36. Based on paragraph 4, it appears that reductionist accounts of causation typically focus on which of the following causes?

A. Social causes, because they are directly related to effects

B. Physiological causes, more assignable to effects, in general

C. Both social and physiological causes as simultaneous causes

D. Either; the point is that reductionist accounts attempt to break down general causes into more specific ones

37. Based on the passage, an assumption made by those who argue against physiological accounts of causation is that:

A. physiological accounts of causation tend to disregard the potential existence of harmful social agents.

B. physiological accounts of causation are often incorrect by neglecting the social causes.

C. social accounts of causation can replace physiological accounts of causation.

D. explanations can be reductionist without being physiological.

38. The author mentions individuals in non-industrialised Marxist countries to make which of the following points?

A. Post-industrial capitalism is not a necessary precondition for tuberculosis.
B. Regardless of one's location, tubercle bacillus bacteria is the actual cause of tuberculosis.
C. Living in an industrialised capitalist country is not a cause of tuberculosis.
D. The best causal explanations are those which specify necessary conditions.

39. The central point of the passage is that:

A. while the social accounts of causation are important, the physiological level provides better causal explanations.
B. though some are suspicious, there are good reasons for including physiological accounts of causation along with social accounts of causation.
C. people arguing against reductionist accounts of causation will most likely endorse the social accounts of causation.
D. people arguing against physiological accounts of causation do not realise their importance.

40. Which of the following is **not** mentioned in the passage as a reason why proximal physiological explanations of causation are as desirable as social ones?

A. They generally share more in an important logical relationship.
B. They are important in determining both causes and potential solutions.
C. They are, in some cases, necessary preconditions for a particular disease.
D. They are more effective in getting at the actual cause of a disease than social explanations of causation.

If time remains, you may re-examine your work. If your allotted time (60 minutes) is complete, please proceed to the Answer Key.

3.8.4 Verbal Reasoning Exercise 2 (Science-based Passages) Answer Key and Worked Solutions

1.	B	9.	D	17.	B	25.	A	33.	D
2.	B	10.	A	18.	D	26.	C	34.	B
3.	A	11.	B	19.	A	27.	D	35.	D
4.	B	12.	A	20.	B	28.	A	36.	B
5.	A	13.	B	21.	B	29.	B	37.	A
6.	C	14.	C	22.	D	30.	C	38.	A
7.	D	15.	D	23.	D	31.	B	39.	B
8.	C	16.	D	24.	B	32.	B	40.	D

1. **Correct Answer: B**
(A), (C), and (D) are all too general and lack the specific focus of the passage, which is adequately expressed in (B).

2. **Correct Answer: B**
(A) and (D), similar to the preceding question are too general. (C) is a statement of policy - marked by the word "should" and a call to action, which is never addressed within the passage. This leaves (B), which possesses the specificity of "purpose" and reflects the passage information, as the best option.

3. **Correct Answer: A**
(D) is too encompassing and not really addressed adequately within the passage. (C) may or may not be true but also never addressed adequately within the passage, except for brief references to clean-up acts. (B) assumes a causal link not adequately established within the passage - there may be other factors involved. The statement needs more support within the passage to qualify as the best answer. (A) is specific enough to qualify as the best choice option in terms of significance and relevance, i.e. one can assume that cyanide toxins will have an "effect" on wildlife within a wetland. This would also be encompassing of the probability or possibility of (B).

4. **Correct Answer: B**
II is never mentioned within the passage while a rescan will confirm that I and III are addressed.

5. **Correct Answer: A**
(D) can quickly be ruled out due to the phrase "green reasoning," which is essentially meaningless. (B) can be ruled out, for there is little evidence which follows a hypothetical line of thought, such as "If this were to happen . . ." or "suppose that . . . then this would follow". (C) can be ruled out because there is no testimony used as support within the passage, such as "noted biologist Dr. Smith" or "the U.S. Geological Survey states that. . ." This leaves (A) as the correct answer, and both examples are used within the passage to support the main idea or thesis.

6. **Correct Answer: C**
This question is answered in paragraph 1: "As social beings, our basic goal is to belong."
(A) Although the passage states that Adlerian Psychology considers people to be choice-making by nature, this is not the most important motive in human interactions.
(B) This is not discussed in the passage.
(D) The passage suggests this should be a goal for many people but not that it is everyone's most basic goal.

7. **Correct Answer: D**
This question asks you to understand the author's definition of a term. Paragraph 3 tells us that the concept involves social involvement and a deep sense of belonging, so the option that involves working with others as equals is the best fit.
(A) Since this choice involves a person acting as an individual and not as a group, it is not the best example.
(B) Since *Gemeinschaftsgefühl* does not involve status-seeking, this is not the best choice.
(C) This choice involves a hierarchical relationship, which may not be conducive to a "deep sense of fellowship".

8. **Correct Answer: C**
This question compares different philosophies. Maslow's ideas emphasise the need for psychological health and overall self-esteem, making it compatible with Adler's interest in the need to avoid feeling inferior.
(A) This choice reduces human behaviour to instinct and impulses.
(B) This contradicts Adlerian psychology, which "holds that human beings are goal-oriented and choice-making by nature, not mechanistically victims of instinct, drives, and environment."
(D) This theory would be in conflict with Adler's beliefs against status-seeking and in favour of community involvement.

9. **Correct Answer: D**
This question asks you what would produce happiness according to Adler's theories. We are told that Adler was the first in the fields of psychiatry and psychology to note the importance of our perceptions and social relationships to our own emotional and physical health and to the health of our families and communities.
(A) The passage implies that this is a large factor in unhappiness but not that it is the greatest factor in mental health.
(B) The passage states that Adler's theories were based on humans making choices, not on innate qualities.
(C) According to Adler, people are not "mechanistically victims of instinct, drives, and environment".

10. **Correct Answer: A**
The answer to this question is answered in paragraph 4: "Adler viewed some behaviour as overcompensation for perceived shortcomings... Some adults act as if they believe, mistakenly, that they belong only when they can control others." This makes (A) the correct answer.
(B) This is the opposite of the best answer choice.
(C) This is not stated in the text.
(D) This is also not supported in the passage.

11. **Correct Answer: B**
This question asks you to think about solutions for the problems that interest Adler. The passage never mentions Adler as having an interest in different personality types or as focussed on work. The best choice is thus (B).
(A) The passage states, "Adlerian therapy helps to 'liberate' clients by helping them move toward a clearer understanding of their unconscious, inferiority-based belief systems."
(C) The passage points out the importance of "nurturing one's innate

abilities to cooperate and contribute through what Adler called the life tasks: work, intimacy, and friendship". Hence, adopting productive ways to develop "one's innate abilities to cooperate and contribute" in order to deal with one's inferiority feelings would be something that will interest Adler. This also includes (D) nurturing relationships with friends and loved ones.

12. Correct Answer: A

All answers (B) (C) and (D) are not "problems" per se, but theoretical issues - worth pursuing in their own terms, but not related to the question. (A) can be inferred to be the "crux" of the problem, indicated by the following passage information: "A central problem of science is how to recognise and define worthwhile subjects for investigation. For one thing, we may be faced with a myriad of opportunities and no means to decide which are going to be fruitful. On the other hand, our environment may limit our ability to recognise scientific problems and possibilities, especially the ones which could lead to significant changes in our understanding."

13. Correct Answer: B

(C) and (D) represent technological and/or verifiability issues in relation to theory, as such both answers can be deduced to be incorrect. (A) knowledge is too broad a subject to be warranted as the correct answer. One can infer (B) criteria - the means by which the two are assessed, to be the best choice option.

14. Correct Answer: C

This detail-oriented question can be answered as (C) from the following passage information: "Polanyi was concerned with what he called the "tacit dimension" in our knowledge. In particular he wished to give proper value to the process of recognising, and making a commitment to, ideas or hypotheses, which may result from a rich understanding and knowledge but cannot be explained by explicit reasoning, in order to carry out the enquiry that will lead to them being more widely understood and accepted."

15. Correct Answer: D

Only I and III can be inferred to be correct in this detail-oriented question, these concepts are within the passage, particularly the discussion in paragraph 3.

16. Correct Answer: D

This is one of the main ideas (the second problem) of paragraph 2 and illustrated and expanded upon in paragraphs 3 and 4.

17. Correct Answer: B

This question requires candidates to find the main idea of the article. The author begins by defining politicisation of science, gives a number of examples in which the Bush administration and others misled the public about significant scientific issues, and concludes that "The issue is far from over." Thus the main point is that (B) this problem is widespread and causes harm.

(A) The author gives multiple examples involving the Bush administration but this may be because they are the most recent at the time of writing, not because the author believes they are the worst.

(C) The author cites examples of conservative-led politicisation but never argues that accurate science typically supports liberal ideas.

(D)The passage suggests that people are sometimes misled by these claims, but this is not the main point.

18. Correct Answer: D

This question requires understanding the contextual meaning of a term used in the passage. This is a comprehension type of question that ACER includes in several passages of their full-length practice exams (the Green and Purple e-books). To determine the correct answer, you need to consider the context of the paragraph or line (specified in the question) in which the term is used. Here, "abstinence-based programmes" is mentioned in the paragraph (paragraph 2) where the author discusses issues involving the politicisation of science and sex education during the Bush administration. The paragraph connects the term with the removal of "information about comprehensive sex education. . . from the CDC's website". This makes (D) the most relevant option.

(A) This context is not discussed in the paragraph.

(B) and (C) would require some extent of outside knowledge about the abstinence-based programme of the Bush administration. This is a knowledge skill that ACER will not test a candidate in the real exam.

19. Correct Answer: A

This question tests your understanding of the author's definition of a term and applying that contextual comprehension to hypothetical scenarios. The passage states: "The politicisation of science is the manipulation of science for political gain. It occurs when government, business, or advocacy groups use legal or economic pressure to influence the findings of scientific research or the way it is disseminated, reported or interpreted." In the given example in option (A), scientific findings are misrepresented in order to support a favoured idea. (A) is the best answer.

(B) Using scientific results to try to influence policy, as in this example, is not what the author means by "politicisation of science".

(C) This is an example of misleading the public, but the issue does not involve science.

(D) Conducting research with a goal in mind is not politicisation, according to the author, as long as the study is conducted and reported properly.

20. Correct Answer: B

This question asks you to seek out statements about the causes and enabling factors of politicisation. The author never suggests that basing political decisions on science is inherently bad but implies that the public should know the real scientific facts.

(A) The author writes approvingly of one such board: "the House Committee on Science and Technology announced the formation of a new subcommittee, the Science Subcommittee on Investigations and Oversight, which handles investigative and oversight activities on matters covering the committee's entire jurisdiction."

(C) This is implied in the discussion of Intelligent Design in paragraph 5: "The overwhelming majority of the scientific community, which supports theories that are testable by experiment or observation, oppose treating ID, which is neither, a scientific theory."

(D) This is implied in the discussion of paragraph 8 of reports being "not released completely to the public, quite possibly due to bipartisan politics."

21. Correct Answer: B

This is another type of question that ACER similarly introduces in their practice e-books in order to assess a candidate's ability to logically deduce the tone or attitude demonstrated in the text. In this particular question, it is crucial to take into account the relevant information provided in the paragraph where Rep. Miller's statement was quoted. In paragraph 8, the author states, "Yet the promised reports were far from adequate (two educational reports) or not released completely to the public, quite possibly due to bipartisan politics and mutual scratch-back negotiations concerning other political agendas." Although the passage author assumes Rep. Miller did not fully deliver what he promised due to politics, there is no evidence stating that Rep. Miller's previous statement was

(D) politically-motivated.

(A) The author is simply saying that "the promised reports were far from adequate... or not released completely to the public". Hence Rep. Miller cannot be inferred to have been lying.

(C) The statement released by Rep. Miller was not part of an advertising.

This leaves (B) as the best answer choice.

22. Correct Answer: D

This question asks you to understand why a particular example of politicisation is considered troubling by the author. The discussion of ID states: "In addition, proponents of 'Intelligent Design' (ID) over 'Evolution' have government-spearheaded efforts to be entered into the public schools and with success. The overwhelming majority of the scientific community, which supports theories that are testable by experiment or observation, oppose treating ID, which is neither a scientific theory." The passage never suggests that simply being controversial is a reason to reject an idea since accurate scientific ideas could also offend people. The correct answer is (D).

(A) The passage gives ID as an example of an idea promoted by a group with a religious message.

(B)This is stated in the claim that "The overwhelming majority of the scientific community, which supports theories that are testable by experiment or observation, oppose treating ID, which is neither a scientific theory."

(C) This is also stated in the passage.

23. Correct Answer: D

This question asks you to seek out and make sense of specific information. The passage states that "the promised reports were far from adequate (two educational reports) or not released completely to the public, quite possibly due to bipartisan politics and mutual scratch-back negotiations concerning other political agendas." Thus it is possible that the political favours were traded to suppress certain information.

(A) The passage never states that the reports were unflattering to anyone.

(B) The passage implies that those concerned did understand their significance.

(C) The reference to mutual scratch-back negotiations suggests that the two US political parties had some power. Also, this answer choice makes specific reference to Republicans and Democrats, which are not the focus of the passage.

24. Correct Answer: B

Options (A) and (D) cannot be correct because epigenetic rules are debated throughout the passage without a conclusion on their existence. Answer choice (C) is wrong because it is not the main idea of the passage to "focus on different behaviours to determine the content of the rules"; rather, the passage mentions specific behaviours to question the concept of such rules in the first place.

While the passage does not mention that the sociobiologists are hasty, the entire passage implies that the notion of epigenetics has been embraced even if there is, as yet, no evidence that it does. Epigenetics is simply an inference that sociobiologists have made since there are several behaviours that are common to most humans.

The passage begins with a premise: genes determine how our brains and neurotransmitters develop. Therefore, according to the sociobiologists, there are common behaviours among humans (fear of the dark, for example). The sociobiologists then jump to include 'morality' in the common behaviours (altruism, for example). From this, the sociobiologists argue that our genes determine our morality. This is a very wide jump from one point to another - it is too sweeping a generalisation. These all mean that the claim was made even before there is evidence for it. That is why it is 'hasty'. Option (B), which is the correct answer, is also found in the second sentence of paragraph 1.

25. Correct Answer: A

Option (C) is true, but that is not the point being made by the author. Option (D) is an opinion, which is not part of the quote. Option (B) cannot be confirmed. This leaves (A) as the best option.

26. Correct Answer: C

In the final paragraph, the author never objects to the linkage between science and morality. He seems to be suspicious at the linkage and then he objects strongly about using genes as a source of a theory of morality. However, he does not say that the genes, which may be linked, should not be sought.

On the other hand, consider the validity of the following statement given the author's assertions: "Genetic discoveries should not be strongly relied on to provide solutions to moral dilemmas." That makes (C) the best answer.

27. Correct Answer: D

Option (D) expresses an idea of Friedrich Nietzsche, which is used in paragraph 4, to extend the author's view that merely knowing the genetic basis of something (or having its origin based on genetics) does not necessarily make the theories on genetics entirely true. This statement in option (D) only extends the main idea of the paragraph, but it is neither supported by an example nor does it serve as an illustration of the author's claim.

(A) This option is supported by the author's discussion in paragraph 1, in which examples of certain phobias are cited. Hence, this is a claim that was supported by examples in the passage.

(B) The claim stated in this option explained in paragraph 2's discussion about altruism. Again, this is a claim that was supported in the passage.

(C) This is a counterclaim cited by the author in paragraph 3. Those who disagree with the theory of "epigenetic rules" highlighted the example of our tendency "to throw spears pointy-end first" as being dictated by human intellect and logic as opposed to being simply a genetic tendency. This counterclaim is, therefore, supported by an illustration in the passage.

28. Correct Answer: A

This question requires differentiating the argument of the author from those of the sources or references cited in his or her article.

The author presents the sociobiologist perspective in the first 2 paragraphs (epigenetic rules, behaviour has a basis in our genes) and then in Paragraph 3, he begins to make his case for environment/experience being understated by epigenetic rules.

If, in the question, it stated that everyone in the world has a near equal fear of snakes, that would support the idea of a human gene (or genes) being responsible for behaviour. However, the question suggests that where you live has an impact on what you fear which is more in line with the (A) author's perspective.

29. Correct Answer: B

This question asks you to carefully read an explanation of an experiment. Paragraph 2 states: "This experiment raised the ethical issue of whether it was morally right for a scientist to encourage people to inflict pain on others for experimental purposes." This suggests that the subjects' actions were unethical because they believed they were doing something cruel even though it was not real and thus the experimenters acted unethically in asking them to do it. This aligns with option (B).

(A) The passage states that there were no actual electric shocks.

(C) Since the passage states that the experimental subjects were fooled, we can guess that the "protesting victims" may have been in on the scheme from the start.

(D) Since the shocks were not real, this would not have been dishonest.

30. Correct Answer: C

This question calls for an understanding of the anti-cloning arguments the passage author presents. Paragraph 2 asks, "How would a cloned child see his individuality after knowing that he was a clone? Wouldn't he feel his individuality as forever compromised?" Since both clones and twins are people who share DNA with someone else, the existence of twins who are content with their identity suggests that this is not necessarily a source of angst.

(A) The passage overall suggests that science must always conform to ethical principles even if it is otherwise beneficial.

(B) The passage suggests that causing suffering to even one person would violate medical ethics.

(D) The passage suggests that cloning is fundamentally different because it duplicates an identity.

31. Correct Answer: B

The passage begins by defining an ethics of science, continues by discussing the type of issues that cause ethical debate, gives examples and concludes that they will be difficult to resolve. Thus the main point is that (B) scientific and medical ethics are contentious.

(A) This is true but a trivial point, not the author's main argument.

(C) The author never suggests that ethics be confined to just philosophical or just medical discussion.

(D) This is not stated in the passage.

32. Correct Answer: B

The answer to this question can be found in paragraph 3: "The argument that ended the debate in the UK leading to the legitimising of such research, up to the 14-day limit, was that a pre-14 day embryo was not in a state to be treated as an individual person since its cells were not differentiated to fulfil specific functions along with the possibility that the embryo was still in a condition to split into two identical twins." Thus (B) the lack of certain basic physiological traits separates these embryos from human beings.

(A) The passage never mentions pain.

(C) The passage does not discuss personality and free will.

(D) This is irrelevant since embryos much older than 14 days are also not viable outside the womb.

33. Correct Answer: D

This type of vocabulary question is common in ACER practice exams. Answering this question requires a reading comprehension skill called contextual reading as discussed in RHSS 3.2.2. Hence, you can answer this question by logically guessing from the context of the last paragraph: "Such assumptions, however, cannot be accepted as axiomatic; they are philosophical issues, of course, but also crucial as pertaining to human life itself." The author is saying they cannot be assumed without debate and reasoning, so (D) "taken for granted" works well.

(A) and (B) are irrelevant to the context of the sentence.

(C) The author is saying that they DO need further elaboration.

34. Correct Answer: B

This question asks you to think about a type of rhetorical device in the passage and its overall effects. Examples include:

- "How would a cloned child see his individuality after knowing that he was a clone?"
- "Wouldn't he feel his individuality as forever compromised?"

- "What if things go awry in the cloning process?"
- "Would that constitute a crime against a human?"
- "Who would be held responsible if things go awry?"

The profusion of questions implies both that there are more of them than people may realise and that using this technology is more difficult than it may seem (for instance, since something could go awry). (B) The reader is prompted to think about the questions and realise that they are difficult to answer.

(A) The passage aims not just to state which questions are unsolved but to make the reader think about why they are unsolved.

(C) Many of the examples do not portray scientists as unethical, so this is not the main point.

(D) The author suggests that these questions do not have easy answers - not that the ethical philosophy behind them is correct.

35. Correct Answer: D

The answer to the question can be deduced from the following: "This idea has its biological correlate in Darwin's theory of natural selection where evolution takes place at the level of the reproduction of individuals in a species."

Option (B) gives the definition of reductionist thinking but it does not state what capitalism and Darwinism have in common - which is, (D) both go down to the level of the individuals.

36. Correct Answer: B

The answer to the question can be deduced from the following:

"We would also be more effective in solving our problems if we moved away from the tendency to focus merely on the proximal physiological causes of disease, for example, focusing on the bacteria or viruses associated with disease instead of social factors."

37. Correct Answer: A

The answer to this question is briefly implied in the last paragraph of the passage: "Short-sighted causal explanation allows for the social structure to go unexamined for its deleterious effects on the community. . ." This makes (B) somewhat inaccurate. At the most, the author would simply consider that focusing on physiological causes alone is "a terribly impoverished way of viewing biology," but not entirely incorrect. After all, "physiological explanations are important in determining the cause and potential solutions."

(C) is out scope.

(D) can be a tempting option. However, this statement would imply that even explanations within a social context is reductionist as well.

38. Correct Answer: A

This is a question of why and then an example is used. The answer to this question can be found in paragraph 6:

"In fact, individuals in the upper class and rural areas, as well as individuals in nonindustrial Marxist countries have also become infected by tubercle bacillus bacteria and come down with tuberculosis. This is not to say that for something to be labeled a cause of disease it must be a necessary condition, but the logical relationship of necessity helps us understand the claim that something is the cause of something else."

(A) is why industrialisation is mentioned at all - to illustrate how it is not required. This is the correct answer.

(B) would be mistakenly selected if one does not get the point of the author.

(C) is the opposite of the point being made.

(D) is a vague and irrelevant choice that could be tempting.

39. Correct Answer: B

Option (C) is found in paragraph 4. It is a true statement, but it is not the main argument of the passage. (D) is slightly discussed in paragraph

5 but it is not a valid argument. (A) is also wrong because the whole passage talks about both social and physiological accounts; not about how one is better than another. This leaves (B) as the correct answer.

The central point of the passage can be followed this way: First, it explains what it means when we say that something causes disease. The passage asserts that when doctors say that bacteria cause disease, the doctor is simply saying that the immediate physiological cause is the presence of the bacteria. It is the most precise and measurable way of finding out what causes disease.

The passage also asserts that these physiological causation do not take into account social agents that may cause disease. Because it is difficult to precisely and accurately pinpoint which social agents cause disease, people are suspicious about social agents causing disease.

40. Correct Answer: D

This question asks you to choose which of the options was NOT mentioned in the passage. Option (D) is the best answer because it states that physiological causes are more effective in determining the actual cause of the disease that social causes. This is NOT mentioned in the passage. What the passage actually states is that we would be more effective if we focussed not only on the physiological causes but also on the social causes.

This part of the passage directly contradicts statement (D):

"We would also be more effective in solving our problems if we moved away from the tendency to focus merely on the proximal physiological causes of disease, for example, focussing on the bacteria or viruses associated with disease instead of social factors."

High-level Importance

SPOILER ALERT ⚠

Gold Standard has cross-referenced the content in this chapter to examples from ACER's official GAMSAT practice materials. It is for you to decide when you want to explore these questions since you may want to preserve some of ACER's materials for timed mock-exam practice.

Examples – Literature and Arts in Medicine or Science - Q30-34, Q59-62 of 5; Philosophy and Science - Q45-48 of 3; Social Science Theories - Q1-6 of 2, Q30-35 and Q45-48 of 3, Q42-45 of 4, Q1-5, Q50-54, Q68-73 of 5; Medical Treatments or Procedures - Q27-32 of 1, Q18-20 of 4, Q50-54, Q55-57 of 5; Medical Ethics - Q18-22 of 3, Q22-26 and Q46-54 of 4. Note that "Q" is followed by the question number, and, for example, "of 1" refers to booklet number 1 which is referenced in the Spoiler Alert table at the end of section RHSS 3.2.4. The 15 full-length HEAPS GAMSAT practice tests (by Gold Standard) include exams that contain specific cross-references to this chapter within the worked solutions.

Chapter Checklist

- ☐ Access your online account to view answers, worked solutions and discussion boards.
- ☐ Complete a maximum of 1 page of notes using symbols/abbreviations to represent the content in the foregoing section. These are your Gold Notes.
- ☐ Consider your options based on your optimal way of learning:
  - ☐ Create your own, tangible study cards or try the free app: Anki.
  - ☐ Record your voice reading your Gold Notes onto your smartphone (MP3s) and listen during exercise, transportation, etc.
  - ☐ Consider reading at least 1 source material every day (e.g., poems of a single author, a synopsis of a novel, an article from a scientific journal that caught your interest, etc.). Note down the main idea or ideas of the piece on your scratch paper. Determine or surmise the author's sentiment or purpose for writing the material.
- ☐ Reassess your schedule for your full-length GAMSAT practice tests: ACER and/or HEAPS exams. Ensure that you have scheduled one full day to complete a practice test and 1-2 days for a thorough assessment of worked solutions while adding to your abbreviated Gold Notes.
- ☐ Reassess your progress in scheduling and/or evaluating stress reduction techniques such as regular exercise (sports), yoga, meditation and/or mindfulness exercises (*see* YouTube for suggestions).

3.8.5 Doctor-Patient Interaction Test

Candidates who have sat recent GAMSAT exams reported having encountered Units with doctor-patient scenarios. Most of the questions in these passage types require candidates to infer tone and purpose in a conversation. Before attempting the following questions, it might be a good idea to revise the discussion and short exercises in RHSS 3.5.5 (Tone Questions).

Please choose the best answer for each question. You have 16 minutes. Please time yourself.

BEGIN ONLY WHEN TIMER IS READY.

Unit 1

Questions 1 - 4

The following passage is an interaction between Emma and her general practitioner about her son James. Emma has brought her son to the doctor because of a rash.

Doctor: Emma, I don't want to alarm you but because of James' rash and how long he's been unwell, I would recommend that you take him to the hospital immediately.

Emma: The hospital? I don't think he's that sick; I thought he'd just need some antibiotics.

Doctor: At the moment, I don't think antibiotics will be helpful for James. Hopefully, all the investigations at the hospital will just be routine and he won't have to be admitted; but we need to be sure.

Emma: I guess we can take him to the hospital. I'll get my husband to drive us when he gets home from work and I've finished doing my errands.

Doctor: Actually, he needs to go as soon as possible. I can arrange for an ambulance to pick him up immediately.

Emma: Ok, if that's what you think is necessary.

1. Which best describes the tone of the doctor in the above statement?

A. Tactful
B. Anxious
C. Incredulous
D. Relaxed

2. Emma's initial reaction to the news about her son can be best described as:

A. confused.
B. incredulous.
C. infuriated.
D. accepting.

3. Consider the following sentence from the given scenario.

Doctor: Emma, I don't want to alarm you but because of James' rash and how long he's been unwell, I would recommend that you take him to the hospital immediately.

What type of response from Emma would the doctor expect at this point in the conversation?

A. Relaxed
B. Concerned
C. Stolid
D. Angry

4. Consider Emma's final statement to the doctor.

Emma: Ok, if that's what you think is necessary.

Emma's final response is best described by which of the following?

A. She is now concerned about her son's health.
B. She doesn't care about what happens to her son.
C. She is annoyed that her plans have been interrupted.
D. She is willing to do what her doctor has recommended.

Unit 2

Questions 5 - 7

An elderly woman is sitting next to a male medical student on a plane as he reads a medical textbook. She notices the textbook and, after realising he is a medical student, she begins to relate concerns about her health. She relates that has fallen twice in the past few months. She continues by telling the student about her multiple surgeries and the significant list of medications. Despite all of this, she claims her GP brushes away her concerns.

5. The woman appears to be:
   A. perturbed.
   B. beside herself.
   C. disturbed.
   D. distraught.

6. The medical student would most likely respond to the woman by:
   A. politely rebuffing the woman, explaining the need to study.
   B. asking her if she could further explain some of her illnesses.
   C. explaining to the woman that many people her age fall down and she should not worry.
   D. None of the above.

7. Near the end of the plane journey, the woman asks the student for advice.

   What is the most appropriate response the student could give?
   A. Ask the woman to repeat herself as he was not sure what the problem could be.
   B. Give her the number of the local hospital and tell her to see a doctor as soon as possible.
   C. Explain that he is a medical student and should not give her any medical advice.
   D. Explain to the woman that many people her age fall down so she should not worry.

Unit 3

Questions 8 - 10

Bacon was inadvertently given to a Muslim patient for his breakfast meal. Due to a previous surgical procedure, the patient did not realise until his father saw the half-eaten meal when he visited him at lunch. The father became very angry and began shouting for a nurse and demanded to see someone in charge.

8. What is the best way to describe the father's reaction?
   A. Appropriate
   B. Audacious
   C. Incensed
   D. Indignant

9. What would be the most appropriate action to take for a healthcare professional who responds first to the patient's father?

A. Acknowledge the mistake and apologise
B. Refer the father to their supervisor
C. Assure the father that the employee responsible will be reprimanded
D. Inform the head nurse and the health workers who distributed the meals

10. Medical students are considered 'part of the hospital' and must be amiable when interacting with patients.

Given the same given scenario, how would a first-year medical student initially respond to the patient's father?

A. Acknowledge the mistake and apologise
B. Guide the father to their supervisor
C. Assure the father that the employee responsible will be made accountable
D. Inform the head nurse and the health workers who distributed the meals

If time remains, you may re-examine your work. If your allotted time (16 minutes) is complete, please proceed to the Answer Key.

3.8.6 Doctor-Patient Interaction Test Answer Key and Worked Solutions

1.	A	**3.**	B	**5.**	A	**7.**	C	**9.**	A
2.	B	**4.**	D	**6.**	D	**8.**	C	**10.**	A

1. **Correct Answer: A**
In this conversation, the doctor is able to make Emma understand the urgency of bringing her son to the hospital by providing medically sound reasons. The doctor remains calm and diplomatic despite insisting that James is brought to the hospital for proper evaluation. This rules out (B) anxious and (C) incredulous as possible options. The doctor cannot be inferred to be (D) relaxed since he continues to urge Emma to act immediately. The best answer is (A).

2. **Correct Answer: B**
Emma's response upon hearing the doctor's advice to bring her son to the hospital can be inferred as that of (B) disbelief. Her statement denotes she expected the doctor to merely prescribe medication for James. If she was confused, she would have asked more clarificatory questions. This makes option (A) incorrect. Her tone changed to being (D) accepting only in the latter part of the conversation. Nothing in the conversation indicates that Emma expressed (C) anger.

3. **Correct Answer: B**
The answer to this question can be deduced from the beginning of the doctor's statement: "I don't want to alarm you". Had the doctor expected Emma to be (A) relaxed or (C) composed, the doctor would have told Emma straight away that James should be admitted to the hospital. On the other hand, expecting someone to get angry would require a different tone such as, "I want you to stay calm".

4. **Correct Answer: D**
Emma's last line implies trust that the doctor will act in the best interest of her son's health. Hence, a tone of (D) willingness can be inferred. Nothing in the statement proves that she was (C) annoyed or (B) did not care. It can be reasonably assumed that she has become (A) concerned, but that is the reason why she was willing to follow the doctor's advice.

5. **Correct Answer: A**
The candidate should identify that the woman in this scenario is feeling anxious (via her concern, relating her multiple surgeries and her significant list of medications). In this instance, the word (A) perturbed (meaning anxious, unsettled or upset) is most analogous. The general behaviour of the woman does not imply she was antsy (agitated or impatient). (C) Disturbed, in this instance, is analogous to upset and does not match the anxiety shown by this woman. Both (B) "beside herself" and (D) "distraught" would imply she is overly sad or angry about her experience and medications rather than anxious and worried.

6. **Correct Answer: D**
It is important for the candidate to remain compassionate as it is obvious the woman is anxious or perturbed. To understand why option (D) is the correct answer, the candidate should know that the best response would be to calm the woman and point her in the direction of a medical professional. A further conversation could explain how getting a second opinion is a great option, and any concerns she has should be raised with a medical professional. This answer shows that (A) rebuffing would be insensitive as the woman is clearly distressed and you could easily point her in the direction of someone who could help her. It could be interesting to (B) hear the woman elaborate on her illnesses; however, this is not the best response as a medical student is not qualified to give any advice, even if it is taken directly from a textbook. Option (C) is true in that many elderly people fall down, but there is definitely cause to worry about her safety. Therefore, (D) none of the given options is correct.

7. **Correct Answer: C**
It is important for candidates to identify that only licensed medical professionals should give medical advice. This makes (C) the correct answer. Following this, option (A) should not be considered as it might encourage the woman to continue asking the medical student for advice on her illnesses. (B) could instil a sense of panic in an already anxious woman and is not correct. (D) As already stated, the woman may have a serious condition that needs attention.

8. **Correct Answer: C**
In this instance, it was clear that the father reacted angrily. It could be said the father acted (A) appropriately to the situation. However, in this instance, the BEST word to describe the father should be analogous to exhibiting anger, which is (C) incensed. (B) An impudent lack of respect could again be argued. However, no direct untoward disrespect shown to any member of the staff is mentioned in the passage. (D) Indignant is close; however, it conveys a more annoyed tone than the anger and passion shown by the father.

9. **Correct Answer: A**
The first and most logical action to take during conflict resolution is to (A) acknowledge the mistake on the part of the hospital staff. Option (B) is a good option and will certainly come later. However, it would still come after apologising. Option (C) would come from someone who manages the ward/hospital. It is not the role of the first responder, which is to calm the aggrieved party and acknowledge the conflict. Option (D), in a similar vein to option (B) will come later. However, the father is of priority and communication with him is most important.

10. **Correct Answer: A**
The best option in this situation is exactly the same as the previous question for similar reasons: the patient needs to be calmed down first. A medical student is part of the hospital, and it would still be appropriate to (A) apologise on behalf of the hospital. Options (B) and (D) would be the ensuing actions while option (C) is wholly inappropriate for a medical student to say.

3.8.7 Poetry Test

Units with poems or song lyrics appear one to three times in Reasoning in Humanities and Social Sciences of the new digital GAMSAT exams. Recent sittings would include Poetry Units that consist of a set of three or more poems sharing a similar subject or theme.

This Poetry mini test is composed of 5 units, each with one poem as the stimulus. They are designed to get you used to interpreting themes, patterns, and symbolisms in poems and songs, among others. If you wish to attempt Poetry Tests with more than one poem in a single set, you may access them in our full-length practice tests.

GAMSAT Poetry Tips:

- Read at least one poem a day.
- Learn common literary devices and symbolisms.
- 3 months before the exam, sit poetry mini tests regularly.
- 4 weeks before the exam, attempt full-length GAMSAT practice tests, in order to get comfortable answering poetry questions in an exam-day format with multiple units covering various topics in Humanities and Social Sciences.

There are 20 questions in this mini test. Please choose the best answer for each question. You have 32 minutes. Please time yourself.

Guide Questions for Understanding Poetry

- What is the central idea of the poem?
- What images are described in the poem?
- How do the images relate to each other?
- Is there an overarching image, character or mood that the poem emphasises? Does it form a unified pattern throughout the poem?

BEGIN ONLY WHEN TIMER IS READY.

Unit 1

Questions 1 - 4

Chemin De Fer

Alone on the railroad track
I walked with pounding heart.
The ties were too close together
or maybe too far apart.

The scenery was impoverished:
scrub-pine and oak; beyond
its mingled gray-green foliage
I saw the little pond

where the dirty old hermit lives,
lie like an old tear
holding onto its injuries
lucidly year after year.

The hermit shot off his shot-gun
and the tree by his cabin shook.
Over the pond went a ripple
the pet hen went chook-chook.

"Love should be put into action!"
Screamed the old hermit.
Across the pond an echo
Tried and tried to confirm it.

Elizabeth Bishop

1. The emotions expressed by the speaker walking with a "pounding heart" (line 2) and the dirty old hermit "holding onto its injuries" (line 11) suggest that:

A. both characters suffer from insecurity.
B. the speaker is in a state of flight while the hermit, of entrapment.
C. both characters are experiencing pain.
D. the speaker's present mood is positive while the hermit's, negative.

2. "Chemin De Fer" is a French word for railroad. The title of the poem and the meaning evoked by the last two lines represent:

A. indifference.
B. an unwelcomed rebound.
C. stagnation.
D. an inescapable cycle.

3. The poet's use of the image of the pond (line 8) and her reference to the echo (lines 19 - 20) imply that:

A. the hermit represents the pond; and the speaker, the echo.
B. both characters similarly feel isolated.
C. the hermit is an outcast and the speaker is a fugitive.
D. the speaker and the hermit represent one and the same person.

4. Which of the following insights about Elizabeth Bishop's poetic style best describe the quality of "Chemin Do Fer"?

A. Too much intellectualisation of the poetic images results to obliquity.
B. Heavily using extended metaphors creates a mask of the poet's persona.
C. Using an outsider's perception to view another outsider's circumstance is an effective means of identifying perceptions and consciousness.
D. To identify one's self as an outcast and to try to live, and love, in two worlds, is to dream of the impossible safe place.

Unit 2

Questions 5 - 7

Driving to Town Late to Mail a Letter

It is a cold and snowy night. The main street is deserted.
The only things moving are swirls of snow.
As I lift the mailbox door, I feel its cold iron.
There is a privacy I love in this snowy night.
Driving around, I will waste more time.

Robert Bly

5. Based on the images described in the first 3 lines, what is the atmosphere of the poem?

A. Melancholic
B. Austere
C. Stark
D. Desolate

6. The irregular rhythm and metre of the poem help create which effect that accurately suggests the poem's overall scenario?
   - **A.** An attempt to break away from monotony
   - **B.** An aimless disposition
   - **C.** A relaxed atmosphere
   - **D.** Disinterest in important matters

7. The last 2 lines of the poem imply that the speaker:
   - **A.** perceives life as lacking in purpose.
   - **B.** considers solitude to be a waste of time.
   - **C.** ends his ambivalent mood with a final choice to "waste more time".
   - **D.** welcomes the chance to commune with nature and the self.

Unit 3

Questions 8 - 12

The Waking

I wake to sleep, and take my waking slow.
I feel my fate in what I cannot fear.
I learn by going where I have to go.

We think by feeling. What is there to know?
I hear my being dance from ear to ear.
I wake to sleep, and take my waking slow.

Of those so close beside me, which are you?
God bless the Ground! I shall walk softly there,
And learn by going where I have to go.

Light takes the Tree; but who can tell us how?
The lowly worm climbs up a winding stair;
I wake to sleep, and take my waking slow.

Great Nature has another thing to do
To you and me, so take the lively air,
And, lovely, learn by going where to go.

This shaking keeps me steady. I should know.
What falls away is always. And is near.
I wake to sleep, and take my waking slow.
I learn by going where I have to go.

Theodore Roethke

8. The line "I wake to sleep, and take my waking slow. . ." has generated various interpretations from several critics, the most predominant of which is in reference to "dying". Which of the following lines would reinforce this interpretation?

- **A.** Light takes the Tree; but who can tell us how?
- **B.** This shaking keeps me steady.
- **C.** Great Nature has another thing to do. . .
- **D.** I learn by going where I have to go.

9. Which tone do the repeating, heavily end-stopped lines of the poem create?

- **A.** Shortness of breath
- **B.** Cycle and Stability
- **C.** Interrupted thoughts
- **D.** Emphasis and Confidence

10. The paradox introduced in the first line is further reinforced in several succeeding lines of the poem (lines 2, 11, 16, 17) in order to:

- **A.** emphasise the contrast between life and death.
- **B.** indicate a peaceful acceptance of the inevitable.
- **C.** illustrate opposing forces in life.
- **D.** reflect the speaker's confusion.

11. Another interpretation of the poem is that the theme revolves around its rejection of the intellect as the way to "enlightenment". What would support this interpretation?

- **A.** The repeated use of words based on feelings rather than reason
- **B.** The poem's constant use of paradoxes
- **C.** The poet's romantic references to Nature
- **D.** The predominance of irrational lines

12. "What falls away is always. And is near" suggests:

- **A.** resignation to one's fate.
- **B.** a fast approaching death.
- **C.** the inseparability of life and death.
- **D.** fear of the uncertain.

High-level Importance

Unit 4

Questions 13 – 16

One Flesh

Lying apart now, each in a separate bed,
He with a book, keeping the light on late,
She like a girl dreaming of childhood,
All men elsewhere - it is as if they wait
Some new event: the book he holds unread,
Her eyes fixed on the shadows overhead.

Tossed up like flotsam from a former passion,
How cool they lie. They hardly ever touch,
Or if they do, it is like a confession
Of having little feeling - or too much.
Chastity faces them, a destination
For which their whole lives were a preparation.

Strangely apart, yet strangely close together,
Silence between them like a thread to hold
And not wind in. And time itself's a feather
Touching them gently. Do they know they're old,
These two who are my father and my mother
Whose fire from which I came, has now grown cold?

Elizabeth Jennings

13. What does "chastity" (line 11) mean in the second stanza?

A. Abstinence
B. Isolation
C. Virtue
D. Mortality

14. The different meanings of "touch" in lines 8 and 16, respectively, equate:

A. truth and evanescence.
B. youth and old age.
C. passion and time.
D. action and imagination.

15. The thread (line 14) signifies:

A. union.
B. spiritual isolation.
C. absence of communication.
D. lifeline.

16. "Flotsam" (line 7) symbolises:

A. spent passion.
B. incapacity.
C. uselessness.
D. deterioration.

Unit 5

Questions 17 - 20

Gift

O my love, what gift of mine
Shall I give you this dawn?
A morning song?
But morning does not last long -
The heat of the sun
Wilts like a flower
And songs that tire
Are done.

O friend, when you come to my gate.
At dusk
What is it you ask?
What shall I bring you?
A light?

A lamp from a secret corner of my silent house?
But will you want to take it with you
Down the crowded street?
Alas,
The wind will blow it out.

Whatever gifts are in my power to give you,
Be they flowers,
Be they gems for your neck
How can they please you
If in time they must surely wither,
Crack,
Lose lustre?
All that my hands can place in yours
Will slip through your fingers
And fall forgotten to the dust
To turn into dust.

High-level Importance

Rather,
When you have leisure,
Wander idly through my garden in spring
And let an unknown, hidden flower's scent startle you
Into sudden wondering-
Let that displaced moment
Be my gift.
Or if, as you peer your way down a shady avenue,
Suddenly, spilled
From the thick gathered tresses of evening
A single shivering fleck of sunset-light stops you,
Turns your daydreams to gold,
Let that light be an innocent
Gift.

Truest treasure is fleeting;
It sparkles for a moment, then goes.
It does not tell its name; its tune
Stops us in our tracks, its dance disappears
At the toss of an anklet
I know no way to it-
No hand, nor word can reach it.
Friend, whatever you take of it,
On your own,
Without asking, without knowing, let that
Be yours.
Anything I can give you is trifling -
Be it a flower, or a song-

Rabindranath Tagore

17. The beginning stanza of the poem depicts:

A. sadness.
B. confusion.
C. a quest.
D. affection.

18. "Displaced moment" (line 35) means:

A. a rare moment.
B. an unexpected chance.
C. a gift.
D. random.

19. "Shady avenue" (line 37) connotes:

A. danger.
B. obstacle.
C. desperation.
D. chaos.

20. The speaker regards the "gift" as something that is:

A. trifling.
B. elusive.
C. spontaneous.
D. surprising.

If time remains, you may re-examine your work. If your allotted time (32 minutes) is complete, please proceed to the Answer Key.

3.8.8 Poetry Test Answer Key and Worked Solutions

1. B	6. B	11. A	16. B
2. D	7. D	12. C	17. D
3. D	8. D	13. D	18. B
4. C	9. B	14. C	19. B
5. D	10. B	15. A	20. C

1. **Correct Answer: B**

This poem is often identified by various critics as one of Bishop's medium in obliquely expressing her own fears and feelings of alienation in reference to her gender identity.

The poet successfully portrays two polarised emotions in this piece: fear resulting to an urge to escape, and frustrations resulting to a refusal to move on. In line 2, being alone on a railroad track and having unstable perceptions of one's path with "ties (being) too close together or... too far apart" connote a sense of danger and of fear. On the other hand, an image of seclusion in the character of the hermit and an echo that bounces back to the hermit's point suggest containment.

This is a "hybrid" type of question that can be answered through a correct interpretation of the emotions depicted in the poem and the evidence found within their contexts.

(A) refers to a likely common feeling experienced by the two characters. The question stem specifically points at two emotions cited in the poem. In (C), pain is apparent in the hermit's character but not necessarily in the speaker's. (D) is a misreading of the tones presented in the poem.

2. **Correct Answer: D**

This question specifically refers to "Chemin De Fer" (railroad) and the last two lines of the poem: "Across the pond an echo / Tried and tried to confirm it." Railroads operating on a recurring schedule is common knowledge. The same recurring action is stated in the repeated sound of the echo. Recurrence denotes a cycle. In addition, the general atmosphere of isolation suggests something inescapable.

(A) is an out-of-context interpretation of the title and the final lines of the poem. (B) is a misinterpretation of the final lines of the poem and is not congruent with a railroad's symbolism. (C) is another aspect of the poem's imagery. However, this is more appropriately represented by the pond – NEITHER the railroad NOR the echo.

3. **Correct Answer: D**

This question requires analysis and relating concepts to the following "pieces of evidence" provided in the poem: (1) Pond contains water. Water mirrors whatever is placed parallel to it; (2) An echo reflects sounds. The poem starts with a premise of escapism. The speaker, therefore, avoids facing his/her own issues by reflecting these on an "invented" character.

(A) is too direct yet does not provide a substantial answer. (B) describes what the two characters may possibly feel but does not answer what the images of the pond and the echo imply. (C) seems plausible; however, this is not the best answer. The question asks: which among the options can identify what is being implied by the poet's use of the image of the pond and her reference to the echo? This requires an answer that will present an insight into the poem's symbolism. (D) is the best option because it offers a considerable interpretation parallel to what the question asks.

4. **Correct Answer: C**

This is an implication question that requires determining two things: the overall idea that the poet tries to communicate in her poem; and, the means or technique that the poet employs in order to get her thoughts across to the readers. This poem speaks about fear and frustration, and flight and confrontation on love. The poet uses images that symbolise the "act of mirroring".

(A) is wrong because the poem is emotionally charged rather than objective or "intellectualised". (B) is halfway true in stating that the extended metaphors hide or indirectly portray the truth. However, the term "persona" distorts the concept of the statement. "Persona" refers to a person's facade, not the inner personality or thinking. (C) is more accurate in presenting an insight into the poem's quality. (D) states the poem's possible theme, NOT an insight about the poem's quality.

5. **Correct Answer: D**

This is a tone question that entails a careful consideration of specific images presented in the poem's first 3 lines. "Swirls of snow" (line 2) calls to mind some sort of a ghost town or deserted place. "Deserted (street)" (line 1) sets such an atmosphere. These two images are powerful enough to connote a desolate – solitary - mood in the first part of the poem.

(A) Although sadness is a possible aspect that comes with a desolate atmosphere, it is not established in the first 3 lines. (B) Austere is wrong. There is nothing severely plain or restrained in the atmosphere that's described in this poem. (C) Stark is a close synonym to the correct answer (desolate). However, stark connotes harshness on top of a barren condition. The line 'There is a privacy I love in this snowy night' does not share this extreme atmosphere.

6. **Correct Answer: B**

This is another tone question that involves recognising the overall attitude or mood of the poem's speaker in relation to the poem's structure. The irregularity in poetic structure combines with the images in depicting a scenario of being adrift or aimless: "swirls of snow" suggests a movement without a definite direction; so does "driving around" with the intention of wasting time.

(A) is an out-of-context interpretation. (C) is a more general view of the poem's atmosphere compared to (B). (D) is not established in the poem. In fact, the speaker has just performed an errand of mailing a letter amid the difficult weather.

7. **Correct Answer: D**

This implication question requires judging the attitude projected by the speaker of the poem in lines 4 and 5. Line 4 reveals the speaker's outlook towards the rather unfriendly weather by stating, "There is a privacy I love in this snowy night." "Wasting time" then, in the poem's essence is not a negative endeavour but an opportunity to enjoy one's private moment.

(A) is an incomplete interpretation of the poem that disregards the speaker's remark in line 4. (B) is a misreading of lines 4 and 5. (C) is wrong because there is no indication in the poem where the speaker is expected to decide or choose.

8. **Correct Answer: D**

In order to understand this seemingly complicated poem, careful consideration of the accompanying details of each line is required. (D) "I learn by going where I have to go" is repeated in the first and last stanzas, as well as every two stanzas in the poem as though it is a reminder of something inevitable - just as death is an inevitable destination. This is, therefore, the correct answer.

(A) Line 10 implies enlightenment rather than death. The image following the line depicts the "lowly worm" climbing to take the light.

(B) Line 16 is a paradox of finding stability out of chaos.

(C) Line 13 is ambiguous. If taken within the context of its stanza, it could mean that the author tells the reader to enjoy what Nature has to offer.

9. **Correct Answer: B**

The lines "I wake to sleep, and take my waking slow" and "I learn by going where I have to go" are alternately repeated in every stanza, either linking the thought of the preceding lines or reasserting a dominant idea of the poem. In effect, this (B) cycle keeps the general context of the poem within the perspectives of these 2 lines.

(A) is not possible because all the lines have complete thoughts. Shortness of breath could have comprised unrelated, broken thoughts. (C) is also wrong because no separate idea is inserted in between the sentences within a single stanza. (D) Emphasis is a possible effect of the repetitions. Confidence, however, is not obvious in the poem.

10. **Correct Answer: B**

In order to arrive at the best answer, the specified lines must first be interpreted.

Line 2: "I feel my fate in what I cannot fear." Instead of fearing the unknown, the line suggests a brave acceptance of one's fate.

Line 11: "The lowly worm climbs up a winding stair." The UPWARD action of climbing to take the light, in contrast to the LOWLY state of a small worm, indicate a slow and quiet determination to elevate ones' self from the "dark" despite the twists ("winding") of life.

Line 16: "This shaking keeps me steady. I should know." Shaking implies the uncertain and unforeseen in life. It can also indicate a sign of a fatal illness. In any case, the speaker expresses a calm ("steady") acknowledgement of such circumstances.

Line 17: "What falls away is always. And is near." This line recognises the fact that "falling away", i.e. opposing forces, is always a part of life.

Lines 2, 11, 16, and 17 altogether convey a positive recognition about certain facts of life. The question calls for a correlation of this shared idea to the first line of the poem, "I wake to sleep, and take my waking slow." Sleeping is as essential as waking, and vice versa. As indicated by the speaker's statement to "take" i.e. "accept" his waking slow, the opposing states of waking and sleeping do not signify a contrast but of inevitability. Hence, it can be inferred that paradoxes are used in the poem to reconcile seemingly unlike states – to be more specific, to accept the inevitable (line 2), the ironies (lines 11 and 17), and the uncertain (line 16) in life.

(A) and (C), therefore, are wrong. (D) is a misinterpretation.

11. **Correct Answer: A**

The answer to this question can be deduced from the following:

"I FEEL my fate in what I cannot FEAR." (line 2);
"We think by FEELING." (line 4);
" LIVELY air" (line 14); and,
"LOVELY, learn by going where to go." (line 15)

Feel, fear, feeling, lively and lovely are subjective words spread in the different stanzas of the poem. In lines 4 and 15, the subjective words are used as a means of thinking and learning, as opposed to using the mind.

(B) is wrong because paradoxes are mainly used in this poem in order to illustrate the innate but inevitable contrast of life, not a rejection of intellect. (C) is debatable because although "Nature" is regarded in romanticism as a contrast to scientific rationalism, "Nature" is usually presented as a work of art itself.
(D) The lines are seemingly irrational at initial reading. However, further analysis reveals that these are meant to show the inherent duality of life.

12. **Correct Answer: C**
"What falls away is always" indicates a condition that lingers. The fact that it "is near" means that it is inescapable too. In other words, death will always come with life.
(A) does not point to the essence of the line being referred in the question. (B) is only applicable to the second statement: "And is near." However, a fast approaching death happens only once, not "always". (D) is not implied in the line or within the context of the stanza.

13. **Correct Answer: A**
The message of this poem is best understood by the logical interpretation of the symbolisms and expressions presented in the poem. These can be inferred from the context of the lines or stanzas specified.
The second stanza alludes to the lack of marital relations between the old couple. The state of having no sexual desire accompanying old age can be said to characterise (A) abstinence.
(B) Isolation is not exactly regarded as something that everyone prepares for in later life. (C) Virtue may be hoped for but this necessitates being morally good or righteous. This is neither implied anywhere in the poem nor is the poem about morality. (D) Mortality does sound like a good option (death being a logical "destination" of human lives), but this will be taking the central theme of the poem out of context and prone to a subjective interpretation. This leaves (A) as the correct answer.

14. **Correct Answer: A**
This question is specifically confined to lines 8 and 16. Respectively, in these lines, touch is likened to a confession and then in the context of time being fleeting. This makes (A) correct.
(C) is literal but does not correctly answer the question. (B) and (D) are mentioned in other parts of the poem but not in response to the lines specified.

15. **Correct Answer: A**
The meaning of this word is taken from the following: "Strangely apart, yet strangely close together, / Silence between them like a thread to hold / And not wind in. And time itself's a feather / Touching them gently." This implies that despite the absence of spoken communication, the couple is still connected by their marital union and by the memories of the time that they have spent together.
(B) and (D) are not implied in the stanza. (C) is a literal reference to the "silence" mentioned in the same line.

16. **Correct Answer: B**
The symbolism of this word can be derived from the following: "Tossed up like flotsam from a former passion, / How cool they lie. They hardly ever touch, / Or if they do, it is like a confession / Of having little feeling - or too much." The general thought of these lines directs to the incapacity of the couple to effectively demonstrate passionate feelings or sexual desires. This makes (B) as the correct answer.
(A) is wrong because the question asks what the word symbolises, not what it means in the context of its sentence or line. (C) would refer to the general function of weak, old people. However, "flotsam" was referred in the poem in relation to passion; hence, (C) is

a remote option. (D) is also wrong because the word is not associated with just a failing capacity but a sexual INcapacity.

17. Correct Answer: D

The reference to a loved one in the beginning line suggests that the poem has an affectionate tone. Therefore, (D) answers this simple inference question. (A) is wrong because the succeeding lines must not be misinterpreted to be depressing but the speaker's way of showing that material things fade through time. (B) is also a misinterpretation. (C) may sound like a possible option because of the line, "what ... / Shall I give you this dawn?" However, the speaker is able to rationalise and answer his own question in the succeeding lines. Therefore, (C) is a weak choice.

18. Correct Answer: B

This is a close reading type of question, which is common in Humanities and Social Sciences. This requires considering the description within the stanza where the word was used in the poem: "...let an unknown, hidden flower's scent startle you" (line 33). This means that a "displaced moment" is unexpected and extraordinary in its occurrence.

Although (A) is true, this answer is encompassed by (B). (C) is what "displaced moment" is being paralleled with by the speaker. The question asks for what the phrase means, NOT to what it is being equated. (D) is not explicitly mentioned in the stanza.

19. Correct Answer: B

This is an inference question that requires contextual interpretation of the stanza. The answer can be deduced from lines 37 to 41. The speaker's reference to a darkness enlightened by a realisation of a dream indicates that "shady avenue" implies the hardships or "obstacles" undergone by a person.

(A) and (C) are not suggested in the stanza. (D) is wrong because the stanza does not mention a circumstance too forceful to constitute chaos.

20. Correct Answer: C

The speaker details his idea of a "gift" in the last stanza. He regards gifts that are material and man-made to be insignificant. Instead, he mentions of "displaced moment" and "whatever you take of it, / on your own, / without asking, without knowing" - things and instances that come at the spur-of-the-moment – to be the "truest treasures". This makes C as the most apt choice.

(A) refers to the material gifts. (B) is wrong because the speaker only mentions the "unexpected" gifts among everyday matters, not those that are hard to find. (D) is a component of being spontaneous, but this choice offers a limited response compared to (C).

SPOILER ALERT

Gold Standard has cross-referenced the content in this chapter to examples from ACER's official GAMSAT practice materials. It is for you to decide when you want to explore these questions since you may want to preserve some of ACER's materials for timed mock-exam practice.

Examples – Poetry units Q22-26 of 1; Q62-64 of 3; Q14-17 of 4; Q9-13 and Q46-49 of 5. Note that "Q" is followed by the question number, and, for example, "of 1" refers to booklet number 1 which is referenced in the Spoiler Alert table at the end of section RHSS 3.2.4. The 15 full-length HEAPS GAMSAT practice tests (by Gold Standard) include exams that contain specific cross-references to this chapter within the worked solutions.

Chapter Checklist

- ☐ Access your online account to view answers, worked solutions and discussion boards.
- ☐ Complete a maximum of 1 page of notes using symbols/abbreviations to represent the content in the foregoing section. These are your Gold Notes.
- ☐ Consider your options based on your optimal way of learning:
    - ☐ Create your own, tangible study cards or try the free app: Anki.
    - ☐ Record your voice reading your Gold Notes onto your smartphone (MP3s) and listen during exercise, transportation, etc.
    - ☐ Consider reading at least 1 source material every day (e.g., poems of a single author, a synopsis of a novel, an article from a scientific journal that caught your interest, etc.). Note down the main idea or ideas of the piece on your scratch paper. Determine or surmise the author's sentiment or purpose for writing the material.
- ☐ Reassess your schedule for your full-length GAMSAT practice tests: ACER and/or HEAPS exams. Ensure that you have scheduled one full day to complete a practice test and 1-2 days for a thorough assessment of worked solutions while adding to your abbreviated Gold Notes.
- ☐ Reassess your progress in scheduling and/or evaluating stress reduction techniques such as regular exercise (sports), yoga, meditation and/or mindfulness exercises (*see* YouTube for suggestions).

High-level Importance

3.8.9 Cartoon Test

High-level Importance

Units with cartoon interpretation usually appear once or twice during the real exam. This mini test presents 11 units with 20 questions. Choose the best answer for each question. You have 32 minutes. Please time yourself accordingly.

BEGIN ONLY WHEN TIMER IS READY.

Unit 1

Questions 1 - 2

Cartoon 1

RUBES® **By Leigh Rubin**

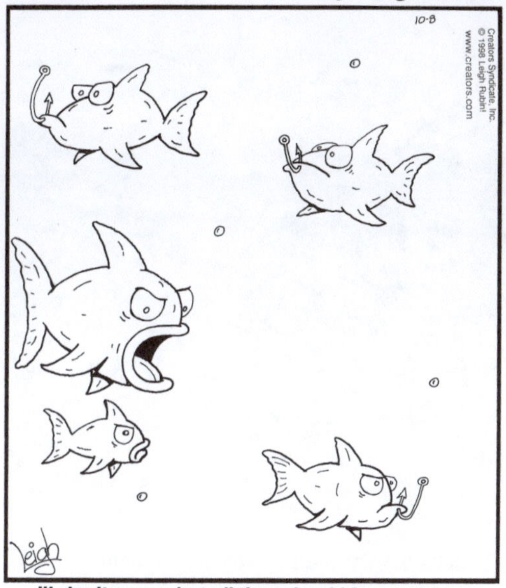

"I don't care what all the other kids are doing, you're *not* getting your lip pierced!"

Reprinted with permission from Creators Syndicate.

1. The humour portrayed in the cartoon mainly relies on:

A. satire.
B. analogy.
C. double meaning.
D. juxtaposition.

2. The dialogue in the cartoon can be paralleled to real-life situations wherein:
- **A.** adolescents tend to imitate fashion trends to the dislike of their parents.
- **B.** parents constantly nag on their children about being too radical.
- **C.** parents and children tend to be at odds when it comes to social conformity.
- **D.** the young generation often ignores the wisdom of the elders.

Unit 2

Questions 3 - 4

For questions 3 and 4, consider the following quotation and analyse the cartoon.

The Internet will help achieve "friction free capitalism" by putting buyer and seller in direct contact and providing more information to both about each other.
Bill Gates

Cartoon 2

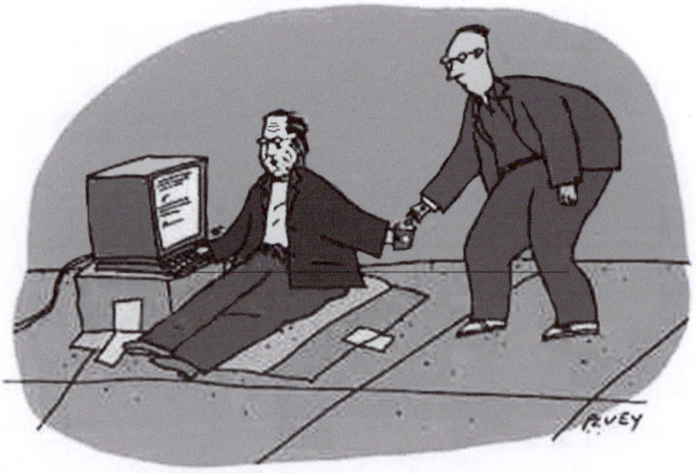

"Thanks pal, let me put you on my mailing list."

Cartoon by P.C. Vey. Reproduced with permission.

3. The statement of Bill Gates is **most** suggestive of:
- **A.** a growth in commerce due to digital technology.
- **B.** a positive development in information systems.
- **C.** good leadership in E-Commerce.
- **D.** the important role of information technology in business trade.

4. This cartoon speaks about:

A. the impoverished working class trying to 'beat the system'.
B. a shift in social stereotypes.
C. the ironic humour of everyday life.
D. the sad plight of homeless people.

Unit 3

Questions 5 - 6

For questions 5 and 6, consider the following comment and analyse the cartoon.

> *Global warming is too serious for the world any longer to ignore its danger or split into opposing factions on it.*
>
> Tony Blair

Cartoon 3

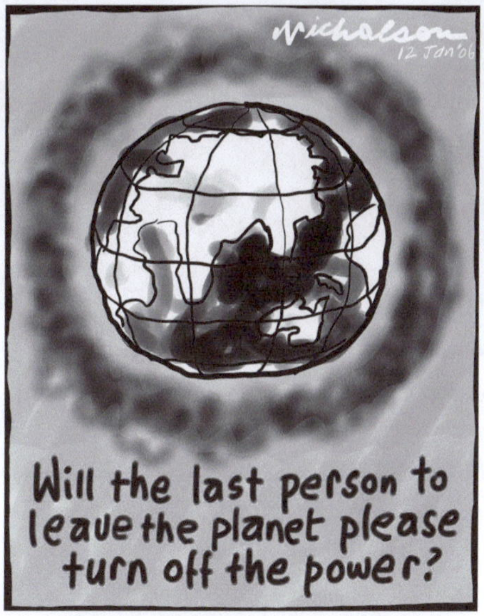

Cartoon by Nicholson from "The Australian" www.nicholsoncartoons.com.au.
Printed with permission.

5. The comment of Tony Blair connotes:

A. an appeal to emotions.
B. an appeal for immediate action.
C. a warning against passivity.
D. a contempt for passivity.

High-level Importance

6. The statement in the cartoon signifies a:

- **A.** positive vision of the future.
- **B.** bleak vision of the future.
- **C.** remote possibility.
- **D.** warning against an impending threat.

Unit 4

Questions 7 - 8

Cartoon 4

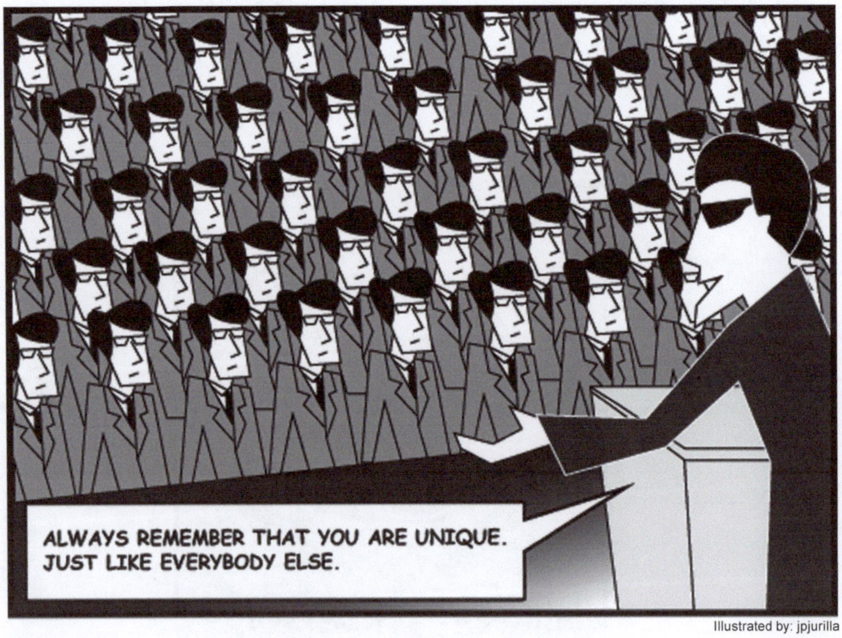

Printed with permission from Jonathan P. Jurilla

7. The cartoon is humorous because:

- **A.** of the analogy between individuality and the audience in the cartoon.
- **B.** of the irony expressed in both the textual and graphical messages.
- **C.** as a matter of fact, individuality is difficult to attain.
- **D.** of the way the message is delivered by the speaker.

8. The cartoon is an example of:
A. graphic art with an erroneous text.
B. a social commentary.
C. irony.
D. a witty remark.

Unit 5

Questions 9 - 11

For questions 9 to 11, consider the following quotation and analyse the cartoon.

A soul mate is someone who has locks that fit our keys, and keys to fit our locks. When we feel safe enough to open the locks, our truest selves step out and we can be completely and honestly who we are; we can be loved for who we are and not for who we're pretending to be. Each unveils the best part of the other. No matter what else goes wrong around us, with that one person we're safe in our own paradise.

Richard Bach

Cartoon 5

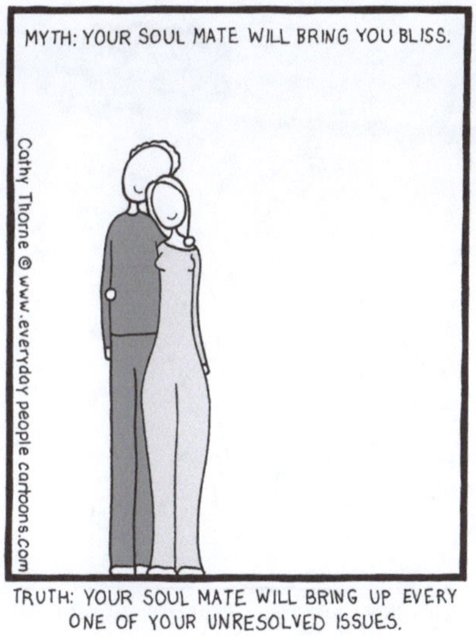

Printed with permission from Cathy Thorne.

9. The statement of Richard Bach describes:
A. a universal truth about love.
B. a lesson learned in finding true love.
C. an aspiration to find true love.
D. an ideal view of romantic love.

10. The statements in the cartoon express:
- **A.** a disbelief in soul mates.
- **B.** a disenchantment with soul mates.
- **C.** the truth about soul mate.
- **D.** an accismus*.

*Accismus: expressing the want of something by denying it.

11. The cartoon could be best described as:
- **A.** a metaphorical illustration of the quotation.
- **B.** a satirical interpretation of the quotation.
- **C.** a trite interpretation of the quotation.
- **D.** an alternative interpretation of the quotation.

Unit 6

Question 12

Cartoon 6

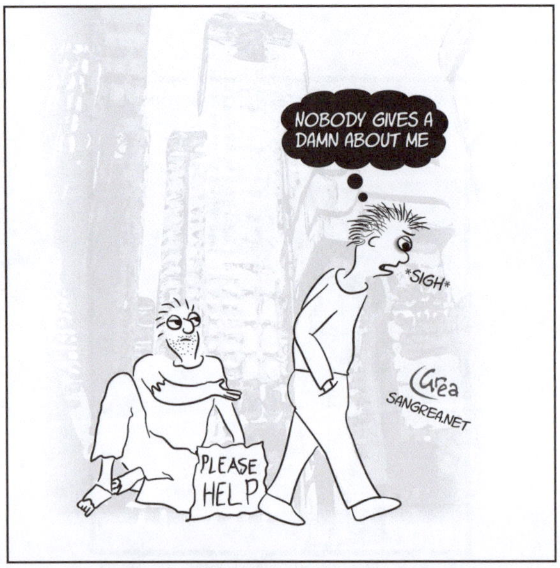

Printed with permission from Grea Korting www.sangrea.net

12. The joke in the cartoon mostly stems from:
- **A.** the similarity in the characters' situations.
- **B.** the juxtaposition of the characters' concerns.
- **C.** the paradox in the speaker's situation.
- **D.** the irony of the characters' situations.

Unit 7

Question 13

The following relates to the importance of good communication skills.

Communication is said to be a vehicle for transferring knowledge and fostering cooperation and understanding in society. Of course, this is not limited to the verbal medium. Nonverbal expressions such as gestures, facial reactions, and signs all form part of the communication process.

Cartoon 7

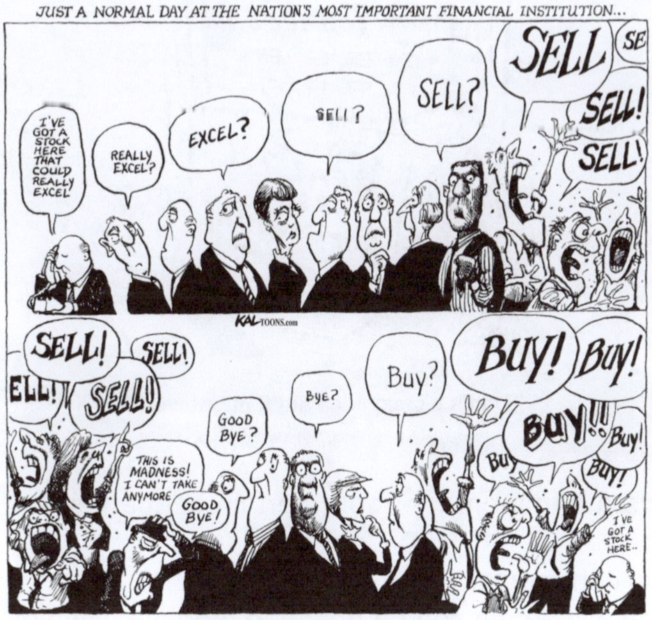

Printed with permission from Kevin Kallaugher.

The following are views of famous writers about communication:

I. I quote others only in order the better to express myself.
- Michel de Montaigne

II. When people talk, listen completely. Most people never listen.
- Ernest Hemingway

III. After all, when you come right down to it, how many people speak the same language even when they speak the same language?
- Russell Hoban

IV. It seemed rather incongruous that in a society of supersophisticated communication, we often suffer from a shortage of listeners.
- Erma Bombeck

13. Which of the four views coincide with the way communication is portrayed in the cartoon?

A. I and II
B. III and IV
C. II, III and IV
D. II and IV

Unit 8

Question 14

Cartoon 8

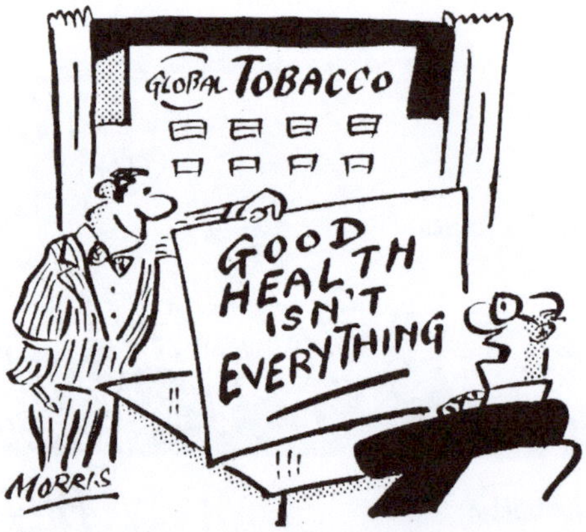

"That's a crazy idea but it might work."

Printed with permission from CartoonStock Ltd.

14. The cartoon reflects a commentary about certain scenarios that resulted from the anti-smoking bans.

Study the following comments:

I. Tobacco companies have sought new and creative ways of getting "around the law" as advertisements have been increasingly regulated with certain bans in print, radio and television media.
II. Health warnings will remain as part of anti-smoking campaigns.
III. Tobacco companies use alternative campaigns that do not necessarily look like tobacco advertisements but have an effect of promoting smoking.
IV. Anti-smoking laws leave tobacco companies with limited marketing alternatives.

Which of these comments would apply to the cartoon?

A. Comment I only
B. Comments II and IV only
C. Comment IV only
D. Comments I and III only

Unit 9

Questions 15 - 16

Cartoon 9

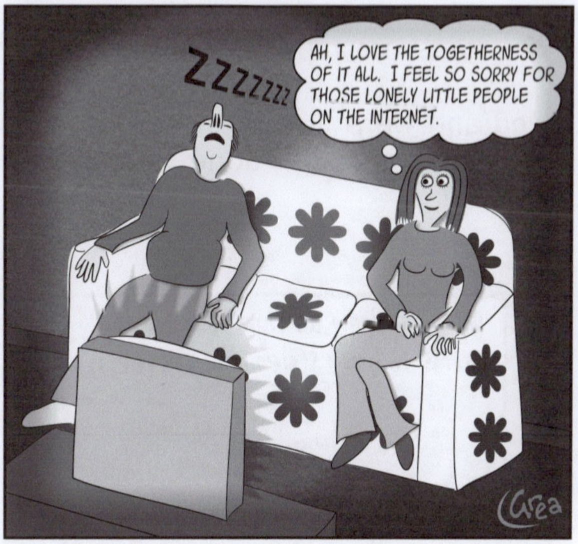

Printed with permission from Grea Korting www.sangrea.net

15. The thought expressed by the wife in the cartoon is an example of:
- **A.** subliminal perception.
- **B.** denial.
- **C.** psychological repression.
- **D.** a metaphor.

16. Based on the cartoon, the best advice on marriage would then be:
- **A.** "A successful marriage requires falling in love many times, always with the same person." (Mignon McLaughlin, The Second Neurotic's Notebook, 1966)
- **B.** "In every marriage more than a week old, there are grounds for divorce. The trick is to find, and continue to find, grounds for marriage." (Robert Anderson, Solitaire & Double Solitaire)
- **C.** "Never feel remorse for what you have thought about your wife; she has thought much worse things about you." (Jean Rostand, Le Mariage, 1927)
- **D.** "I have learned that only two things are necessary to keep one's wife happy. First, let her think she's having her own way. And second, let her have it." (Lyndon B. Johnson)

Unit 10

Questions 17 - 18

In February 2008, former Prime Minister Kevin Rudd read an apology that particularly addressed the "stolen generations" of Aborigines in Australia. Part of the momentous speech was the Parliament's recognition that the indigenous people were indeed mistreated in the past, and that the families suffered severe impacts from the forced removal of the children.

Compensation claims followed and were filed in the courts. However, not all claims were granted because many of the removals were done with consent and in accordance with specific legal acts of the Australian law.

Cartoon 10

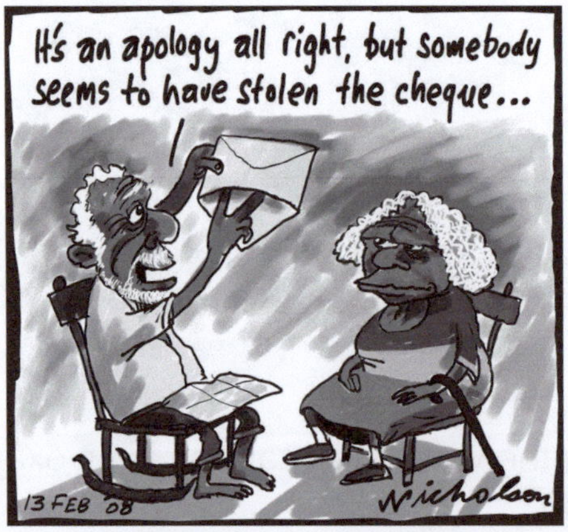

Cartoon by Nicholson from "The Australian" www.nicholsoncartoons.com.au.
Printed with permission.

17. The statement of the speaker in the cartoon:

- **A.** shows that the Aborigines doubted the sincerity of the government's apology.
- **B.** stresses that the Aborigines should be entitled to monetary compensation from the government.
- **C.** shows that some Aborigines possibly did not understand the legal conditions of deserving a payout.
- **D.** stresses that the Aborigines expected compensation to accompany the verbal apology.

18. The word "apology" is used in the cartoon to equate:

- **A.** hypocrisy.
- **B.** vindication.
- **C.** indemnity
- **D.** profit.

Unit 11

Questions 19 - 20

Cartoon 11

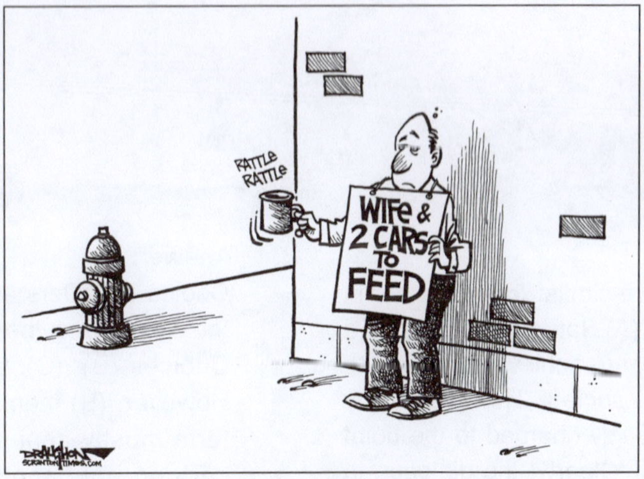

Printed with permission.
(Copyright 2004) Dennis Draughon & The Scranton Times (PA)

19. The cartoon is a reaction to:

A. an economic depression.
B. the unbearable rising prices of petrol.
C. a pretentious lifestyle.
D. social indifference towards the needy.

20. The type of humour found in the cartoon is:

A. a pastiche.
B. an understatement.
C. a parody.
D. a hyperbole.

If time remains, you may re-examine your work. If your allotted time (32 minutes) is complete, please proceed to the Answer Key.

High-level Importance

3.8.10 Cartoon Test Answer Key and Worked Solutions

1.	C	**6.**	D	**11.**	B	**16.**	B
2.	C	**7.**	B	**12.**	D	**17.**	C
3.	D	**8.**	C	**13.**	C	**18.**	C
4.	B	**9.**	D	**14.**	D	**19.**	A
5.	B	**10.**	B	**15.**	B	**20.**	D

1. **Answer: C**

Choices (A) and (D) are similar to each other in their use of contrasts. (A) Satire uses irony as a form of contrast in order to achieve humour with the intent of criticising society. However, irony in satires must be strongly charged to the point of being socio-political. Clearly, the dialogue in the cartoon merely connotes a joke on everyday family life issues.

(D) A juxtaposition is also a form of contrast by placing two elements, which could be objects or texts in an art form, next to each other. In the cartoon, the parent-fish is portrayed to be asserting a parental rule against the child-fish who has already committed the "violation" of this same rule. It would, then, seem that the possible answer to this question would be (D). However, while there is a clear contrast here, another option – (C) – also poses a more appropriate representation of the cartoon's humour.

(C) The cartoon can be interpreted as either a joke about the plight of fishes or as a creative comparison of parent-child conflict in real-life. (C) then becomes the best choice of answer.

(B) An analogy must be expressed in a statement that compares two things. For example, "Her face was a perfect oval, like a circle that had its two sides gently compressed by a ThighMaster." The dialogue in the cartoon does not come close to this form of humour.

2. **Answer: C**

Choice (A) offers a literal interpretation of what the cartoon may be trying to portray.

Choices (B), (C), and (D) are closely similar. However, (B) mentions the word "radical". The term mostly connotes political leanings. The cartoon only shows a fashion trend among youngsters. (D) requires a much profound dialogue or illustration. The best choice is (C) because it embraces a more general interpretation of both the text and the cartoon illustration by using the term "social conformity".

3. **Answer: D**

Although choices (A), (B), and (D) all have something to do with information or identity management, (D) makes an inclusion of the effect of information technology on businesses. Bill Gates' quote uses the term buyer and seller, and these are clearly common terms used on businesses. (C) merely speaks of Bill Gates' status in the internet industry.

4. **Answer: B**

The cartoon satirises a reversal of attitudes and a duality of roles between the beggar and the middle class. In a way, the cartoon does distort the way society generally perceives these two stereotypes. The correct answer is (B).

(A) is easily negated as the correct answer

because, as already mentioned, the cartoon tends to create a duality of roles between a beggar (i.e. accepts a donation) and a member of the working class (i.e. wears an office suit). One couldn't really tell for sure unless the cartoon would be given a literal interpretation.
(C) The cartoon may be portraying an "everyday life" scenario, but the joke doesn't necessarily qualify as an irony of daily life.
(D) There is nothing sad about a homeless beggar who can afford a computer!

5. **Answer: B**
"Too serious for the world any longer to ignore" provides the clue that the comment is not just a statement of (C) warning or (D) opinion but a call for (B) urgency of action. (A) would be a contentious choice.

6. **Answer: D**
(A) is wrong because the cartoon shows the earth on its final days. "The last person to leave the planet" suggests an exodus, which is not exactly a positive thing. (B) Although the cartoon projects humour and witticism, the idea being hinted is rather unwelcoming and terrifying. The statement likewise requests an involvement ("please turn off the power") from the reader ("the last person"), this makes the cartoon, not just a mere presentation of the artist's vision of the future but, more of a (D) warning of a fast coming reality. In other words, option (D) includes the idea in option (B). (C) The accompanying quotation provides the idea of a serious threat or reality, not an impossibility.

7. **Answer: B**
Answering this question requires evaluating the relevance of the text to the graphical illustration. (A) and (D) mislead the examinee to pay primary attention to the image. (C) is a profound interpretation of the cartoon but it is not the device used to make the cartoon humorous. This leaves (B) as the best answer.

8. **Answer: C**
(A) and (B) are the farthest choices because no obvious errors in spelling and grammar can be found nor is there any reference to social or political justice.
(D) The cartoon is more sarcastic than witty.
(C) is the best choice because both the illustration and textual message express subtle mockery and contrasts.

9. **Answer: D**
The quotation simply describes the author's model of a compatible partner in a relationship referred to as a soul mate. "Soul mates" are what many hope to find as expressed in (C). However, the kind of relationship described in the quotation does not always apply to every relationship. Therefore, it is not (A) a universal truth. Obviously, it is not (B) a lesson or wisdom being imparted either. This leaves (D) as the best answer.

10. **Answer: B**
(A) is incorrect as the cartoon acknowledges the existence of soul mates. The second statement, "Your soul mate will bring up every one of your unresolved issues", is just the artist's opinion about soul mates - not a (C) universal truth. (D) is a red herring – there is no evidence to suggest the author of the cartoon/statements is demonstrating a desire for a soul mate via repression. Therefore, (B) is the correct answer.
A little more about answer choice (D): do not expect to find a definition among answer choices during the real GAMSAT, nor during your practice full-length exams. We were just trying to be polite during your training!

11. Answer: B

Since the cartoon portrays an opposite view of the quotation, (A) and (D) can be eliminated from the choices. (B) Taking the quotation into context, it should be noted that there is mention of the line: "Each unveils the best part of the other." One should recall that satire uses humour by highlighting the irony or contrast of a situation or, in this case, the quotation. This is the correct answer. (C) is quite subjective depending on the reader's point of view.

12. Answer: D

The cartoon shows both a (A) similarity and (B) a contrast between the beggar and the passerby. Both characters are in a depressed situation. The beggar seeks financial help yet the passerby overlooked his plight. Ironically, the passerby expresses a need for emotional attention and feels too aggrieved by his own problem that he fails to see the beggar's worse condition. Therefore, the answer is (D) as it encompasses choices (A) and (B). (C) is a ruse: the paradox would have applied to the two characters' situations - not in the speaker's situation.

13. Answer: C

The cartoon is about the distortion of information as words get passed on to the next receiver. In general, the cartoon depicts miscommunication and its source is a failure to listen fully. Quote I is about improving one's communication skills through imitating others. Quote II is an advice to listen and focus as poor listening can be a cause of miscommunication. Quote III implies that miscommunication is common even among people who speak the same language - they don't listen to each other. Quote IV also implies miscommunication even with advanced technology - again, the source is not listening. Choice (C) is the correct answer.

14. Answer: D

Comment I: The line, "That's a crazy idea but it might work", implies entertaining an idea that has not been thought of before – therefore new and creative - but is hoped to pass a certain scrutiny (e.g., an anti-smoking regulation).

Comment II: "Good health isn't everything" is not a health warning.

Comment III: "Good health isn't everything" is another way of saying that there are benefits in vices that cannot be found in a healthy lifestyle. In a way, this is the kind of advertisement described in Comment III.

Comment IV: The cartoon shows a presentation of a novel idea in an advertising campaign. This doesn't show a limitation of options.

15. Answer: B

Of the four choices, (D) metaphor is the easiest to eliminate. A metaphor is an analogy or a parallelism of the resemblance of two things. The statement of the wife expresses a contrast between her situation and those of "the people on the internet".

(A) Subliminal perception requires a stimulus that is unnoticeable but perceived anyway. In the illustration, the wife may look like she doesn't notice her husband falling asleep, but her thoughts in the cartoon tell that she chooses not to recognise it either.

(B) Denial and (C) repression are both forms of defence mechanism. Their main difference is that denial is a refusal to accept a pressing or unbearable problem while repression, against a desire that might result in a problem or cause suffering if that desire is satisfied. The wife is clearly refusing to recognise a lack of "together"-ness with her husband despite spending their time in the same place.

16. Answer: B

(A) can be easily confused as the correct answer. The advice would relate more to extra-marital temptations as opposed to falling in love "with the same person". This situation is not illustrated in the cartoons.

(C) proposes an advice from a husband's standpoint only. The cartoon, however, presents only the wife's perspectives.

(D) This cartoon does not depict a power struggle between husband and wife. Hence, advice (D) is not applicable.

This leaves (B) as the best answer: the wife is finding a way to cope - albeit in an unfavourable light - with their failing communication.

17. Answer: C

(A) The line "It's an apology all right..." indicates that the speaker does acknowledge the apology. What he is only suspicious of is having been cheated in the monetary proceeds due him.

(B) This tone of suspicion in the speaker's statement, however, does not necessarily echo an assertion or a call to grant the compensation.

(C) What can be conveyed from the cartoon is the speaker's expectation of receiving some monetary benefit. This expectation hence illustrates his misunderstanding that all Aborigines will receive a claim. As stated in the descriptive paragraph, NOT ALL Aborigines were granted a payout because others were taken into government guardianship under reasonable circumstances.

(D) Indeed, the cartoon clearly implies that the Aborigines expected to be automatically compensated. This expectation, therefore, highlights the reason why (C) is the correct answer.

18. Answer: C

(A) is not implied anywhere in the cartoon. (B) and (D) sound plausible but not accurate enough in relation to the graphic illustration as well as to the given descriptive paragraph. (C) Indemnity refers to a payment made to someone in order to compensate for damages. This is indicated by the speaker's immediate reaction upon receiving an envelope.

19. Answer: A

While there is an absence of sympathisers and donors in the cartoon, such lack fails to show a discernible portrayal of social indifference either. (D) can be therefore eliminated as the answer.

Having two cars indeed speaks of a high-profiled lifestyle. However, resorting to begging does not necessarily show pretence as it does a decline in one's financial state. Therefore, (C) is not a definite answer.

The cartoon indeed shows either poverty or economic scarcity. The sign bearing the words "2 cars to feed" specifically pinpoints the cause of poverty. (B) The context of rising petrol prices is a little oblique. The correct answer is thus (A) - economic depression.

20. Answer: D

(A) Pastiche is an imitation of another work of art, which is aimed at exalting the original work. The cartoon is not taken from a famous work. Hence, it does not qualify for a pastiche.

(B) An understatement is an extreme diminution of an otherwise important characteristic or topic in order to achieve humour. The cartoon does not reduce the problem implied by the cartoon but rather exaggerates it. A hyperbole exactly does that. The answer is (D).

(C) is wrong because parody is a form of imitation with the intention to mock the original work. This cartoon clearly doesn't do that.

High-level Importance

SPOILER ALERT

Gold Standard has cross-referenced the content in this chapter to examples from ACER's official GAMSAT practice materials. It is for you to decide when you want to explore these questions since you may want to preserve some of ACER's materials for timed mock-exam practice.

Examples – Cartoon units Q11-12 and Q61 of 3; Q65 of 4; Q29 and Q58 of 5. Note that "Q" is followed by the question number, and, for example, "of 1" refers to booklet number 1 which is referenced in the Spoiler Alert table at the end of section RHSS 3.2.4. The 15 full-length HEAPS GAMSAT practice tests (by Gold Standard) include exams that contain specific cross-references to this chapter within the worked solutions.

Chapter Checklist

- ☐ Access your online account to view answers, worked solutions and discussion boards.
- ☐ Complete a maximum of 1 page of notes using symbols/abbreviations to represent the content in the foregoing section. These are your Gold Notes.
- ☐ Consider your options based on your optimal way of learning:
  - ☐ Create your own, tangible study cards or try the free app: Anki.
  - ☐ Record your voice reading your Gold Notes onto your smartphone (MP3s) and listen during exercise, transportation, etc.
  - ☐ Consider reading at least 1 source material every day (e.g., poems of a single author, a synopsis of a novel, an article from a scientific journal that caught your interest, etc.). Note down the main idea or ideas of the piece on your scratch paper. Determine or surmise the author's sentiment or purpose for writing the material.
- ☐ Reassess your schedule for your full-length GAMSAT practice tests: ACER and/or HEAPS exams. Ensure that you have scheduled one full day to complete a practice test and 1-2 days for a thorough assessment of worked solutions while adding to your abbreviated Gold Notes.
- ☐ Reassess your progress in scheduling and/or evaluating stress reduction techniques such as regular exercise (sports), yoga, meditation and/or mindfulness exercises (*see* YouTube for suggestions).

3.8.11 Graphs and Tables Test

The following mini test aims to help you focus on interpreting graphs and tables. These types of stimuli usually appear in one to three Reasoning in Humanities and Social Sciences (RHSS) Units of the GAMSAT.

One of the initial steps in understanding graphs and tables is studying from the maths chapters of the Gold Standard GAMSAT Masters Series Maths and Physics book. Maths is the basis of graphs and tables and must be understood before moving on to GAMSAT-level practice.

With respect to graphs and tables, the difference between RHSS and GAMSAT Sciences is that RHSS graphs and tables' questions are heavily based on qualitative data gathered from social science research (for example, social values and preferences, marriage systems) or theories (for example, socialism, evolution). Knowing what each type of diagram, graph, flowchart, table, and quadrant is used for in social science research can prove beneficial in your preparation.

There are 6 units with 20 questions in this mini test. Please choose the best answer for each question. You have 32 minutes. Please time yourself.

BEGIN ONLY WHEN TIMER IS READY.

Unit 1

Questions 1 - 4

Study the following abstract on medical consultation and the computer, and the accompanying consultation (hermeneutic) circle.

Abstract

Objective: Studies of the doctor–patient relationship have focussed on the elaboration of power and/or authority using a range of techniques to study the encounter between doctor and patient. The widespread adoption of computers by doctors brings a third party into the consultation. While there has been some research into the way doctors view and manage this new relationship, the behaviour of patients in response to the computer is rarely studied. In this paper, the authors use Goffman's dramaturgy (theatrical approach: scene, actor, stage, script, act) to explore patients' approaches to the doctor's computer in the consultation and its influence on the patient–doctor relationship.

Design: Observational study of Australian general practice. 141 consultations from 20 general practitioners were videotaped and analysed using a **hermeneutic framework.***

Results: Patients negotiated the relationship between themselves, the doctor, and the computer demonstrating two themes: dyadic (dealing primarily with the doctor) or triadic (dealing with both computer and doctor). Patients used three signalling behaviours in relation to the computer on the doctor's desk (screen watching, screen ignoring, and screen excluding) to influence the behaviour of the doctor. Patients were able to draw the doctor to the computer and used the computer to challenge the doctor's statements.

Conclusion: This study demonstrates that in consultations where doctors use computers, the computer can legitimately be regarded as part of a triadic relationship. Routine use of computers in the consultation changes the doctor–patient relationship and is altering the distribution of power and authority between doctor and patient.

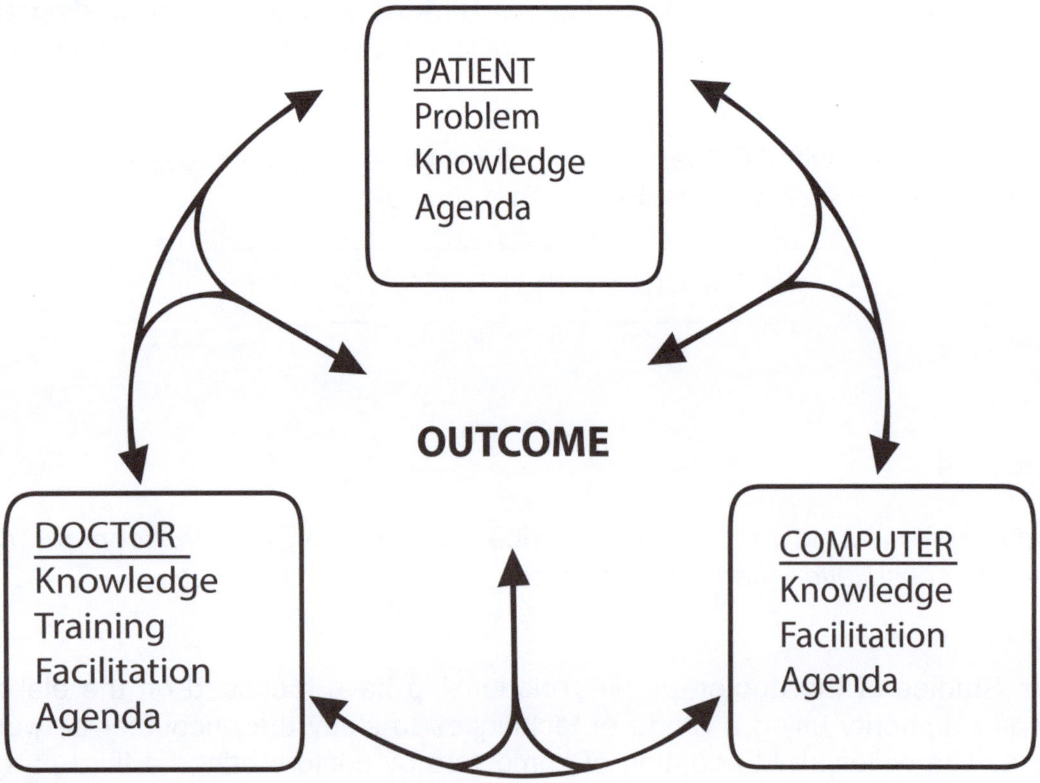

***Hermeneutics** is an old term which refers to the interpretation of biblical, literary, and mythical texts. This process of interpretation (assigning meaning) gathered more momentum in philosophical and social science studies particularly, as to how meaning is developed between the text and the subject – that each mutually defines the other. In as much as we question a given text, it will question or influence us in a co-creation of meaning.*

1. The main focus of the study is:
   - **A.** to document the influence of the computer on the dyadic patient-doctor relationship.
   - **B.** to understand the patient's influence on the doctor's use of the computer in medical consultations.
   - **C.** to explore the patient's behaviour in response to the influence of doctors' use of a computer.
   - **D.** to assess the use of computers in the triadic doctor-patient-computer relationship.

2. Based on the given textual and graphical information, which statement can be said to be the **least** congruent with the meaning of "hermeneutic"?
   - **A.** The use of a computer in consultations transforms doctor-patient relationships and interactions.
   - **B.** The outcome of the consultation is created by mutual interactions between doctor, patient, and the use of a computer.
   - **C.** The patient's perception of the doctor-computer usage influences the outcome of the consultation.
   - **D.** Doctor-patient relationships and interactions are facilitated by a computer in the consultation.

3. The commentary and graph imply that interactions between patient, doctor, and computer comprise a:
   - **A** group relationship with a mutual definition.
   - **B.** triadic relationship with mutual facilitation.
   - **C.** dyadic relationship with a mutual agenda.
   - **D.** processual relationship with mutual knowledge.

4. The metaphor used to approach this research is a:
   - **A.** network.
   - **B.** theatre.
   - **C.** system.
   - **D.** machine.

High-level Importance

Unit 2

Questions 5 - 8

When viewing the chart below, assume that the first score (Judge's) is correct. ***There are errors in the chart in the other ordinal scores.*** *First, find the inconsistencies in the scores to answer the questions.*

CHART (with errors)

	Judge's score *x*	**Score minus 8** *x-8*	**Tripled score** *3x*	**Cubed score** x^3
Alice's cooking ability	10	2	300	1000
Bob's cooking ability	9	1	27	792
Claire's cooking ability	8.5	0.5	25.5	614.125
Dana's cooking ability	8	0	24	521
Edgar's cooking ability	5	3	15	150

5. From the cooks in the chart, who has a correct score in all representational summaries?

A. Edgar
B. Bob
C. Dana
D. Claire

6. The order of the scores, if calculated correctly, can be described to decrease:

A. steadily.
B. exponentially.
C. parsimoniously.
D. regressively.

7. If there were any discrepancies in the tripled score, and they were corrected, the average correct tripled score would be:

A. 24.3
B. 135.3
C. 13.53
D. 23.4

8. What would be the cubed score of the average judge's score?

A. 664.125
B. 531.441
C. 596.025
D. 614.125

Unit 3

Questions 9 - 11

The following are charts measuring oil production and consumption from the years of 1990 – 2009 for both countries: Australia and the U.K. Take note that certain numerical estimates or assumptions are listed below the graphical representations. Study these carefully for certain questions will be based on these estimates.

Australia and UK Oil Production and Consumption

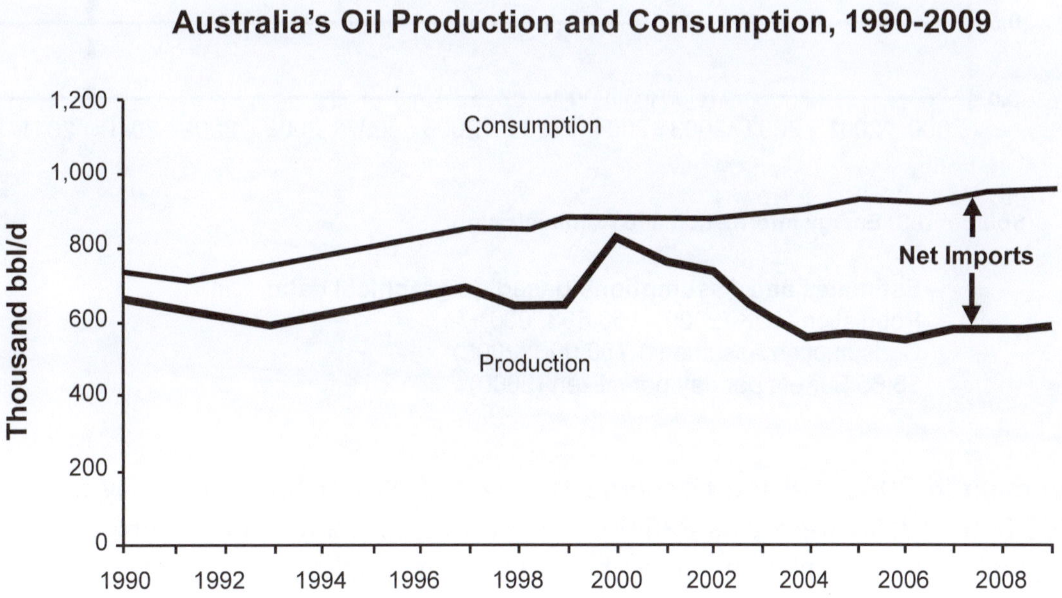

Source: EIA

bbl/d = barrels per day

Estimates and assumptions based on graphical data:
Population – Australia (2000) – 19,153,000 +/-
Consumption Assumed 820,000 (2000)
23.35 barrels per day per citizen (2000)

High-level Importance

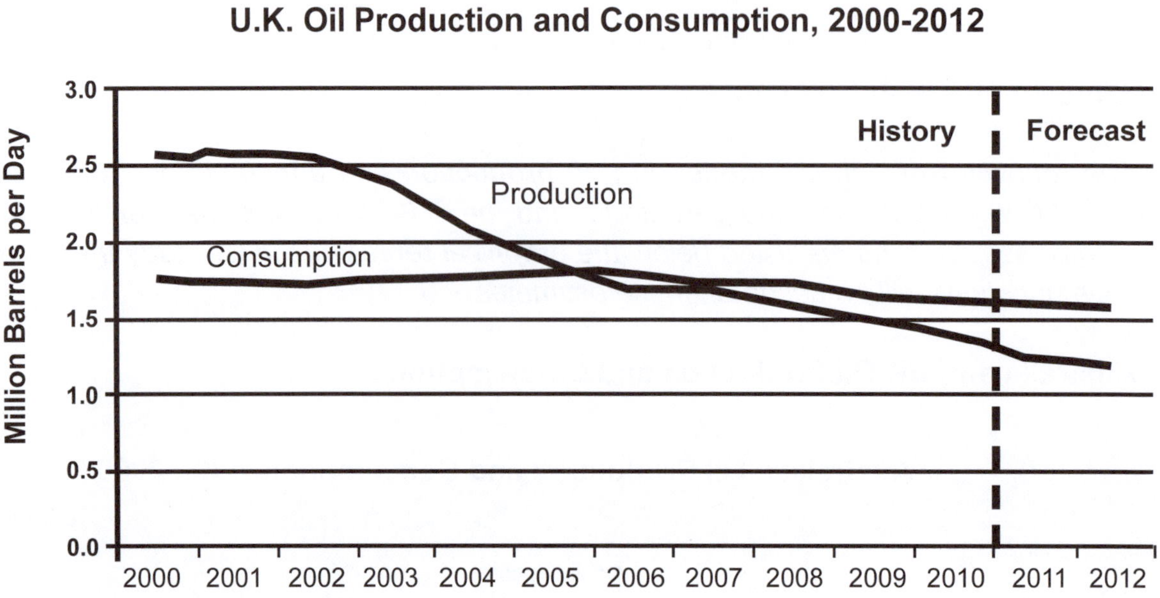

Source: U.S. Energy Information and Administration

Estimates and Assumptions based on graphical data:
Population – UK (2000) – 58,893, 000 +/-
Consumption Assumed 1,750,000 (2000)
33.65 Barrels per day per citizen (2000)

9. Assuming in 2000 that the consumption level of oil per barrel per day for the UK was 1,750,000 and Australia was 820,000, based on the population for that year, what is the rough difference of bbl/d per citizen between each country in that year?

A. 33 **C.** 10
B. 23 **D.** 13

10. The net imports in Australia in 2008 were roughly:

A. 300,000 bbl/d. **C.** 350,000 bbl/d.
B. 400,000 bbl/d. **D.** 450,000 bbl/d.

11. What has been the most consistent variable from both graphs?

A. Production **C.** Consumption
B. Net Imports **D.** Barrels per day

Unit 4

Questions 12 – 15

Carefully read the following commentary and study the accompanying graph.

The PRECEDE-PROCEED planning system or framework is from the National Cancer Institute for communication strategies in health education.

Once health communications planners identify a health problem, they can use a planning framework such as the two described: social marketing and PRECEDE-PROCEED. These planning systems can help identify the social science theories most appropriate for understanding the problem or situation. Thus planners use the theories and models described below within the construct of a planning framework. Using planning systems like social marketing and PRECEDE-PROCEED increases the odds of program success by examining health and behaviour at multiple levels. Planning system perspectives emphasise changing people, their environment, or both.

The PRECEDE-PROCEED framework is an approach to planning that examines the factors contributing to behaviour change. These include:

- Predisposing factors - the individual's knowledge, attitudes, behaviour, beliefs, and values before intervention that affect willingness to change
- Enabling factors - factors in the environment or community of an individual that facilitate or present obstacles to change
- Reinforcing factors - the positive or negative effects of adopting the behaviour (including social support) that influence continuing the behaviour

These factors require that individuals be considered in the context of their community and social structures, and not in isolation, when planning communication or health education strategies.

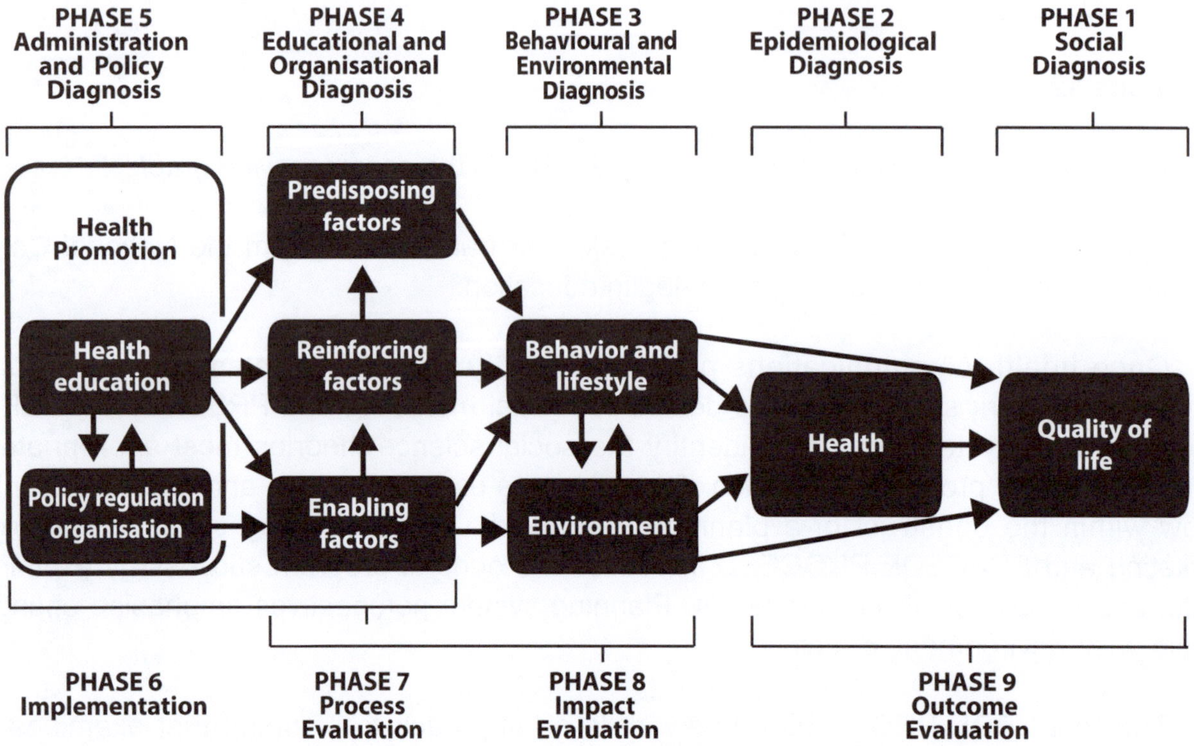

12. The most crucial phases as illustrated in the diagram are phases:

- **A.** 3 and 8.
- **B.** 4 and 7.
- **C.** 5 and 6.
- **D.** 1 and 5.

13. How are phases 3 and 8 related (Behavioural and Environmental Diagnosis and Impact Evaluation, respectively)?

- **A.** Through predisposing, reinforcing and enabling factors
- **B.** Through process evaluation and educational diagnosis
- **C.** Through examining impact evaluation and behavioural/environmental diagnosis
- **D.** Through implementation of the process and epidemiological diagnosis

14. The relationship between phases 5 and 6 can be described as:

- **A.** linear orientation.
- **B.** mutual reciprocity.
- **C.** branching influence.
- **D.** symbiotic or commensal.

15. Based on the information from the text and diagram, why are the three factors considerably important?

A. They are the foundational basis for behavioural change.
B. They are interlinked with impact modification.
C. They are the hub of activity within the graph itself.
D. They are the required phase or level for changes in administration and policy.

Unit 5

Questions 16 - 17

Venn diagrams or set diagrams are diagrams that show all possible logical relations between finite collections of sets (aggregation of things). Venn diagrams were conceived around 1880 by John Venn. They are used to teach elementary set theory, as well as illustrate simple set relationships in probability, logic, statistics, linguistics and computer science. The number of shared areas, according to symbolic logic, is represented by n. These shared areas are logical connections.

Intersections of the Greek, Russian, and English Alphabets –Venn Diagram.

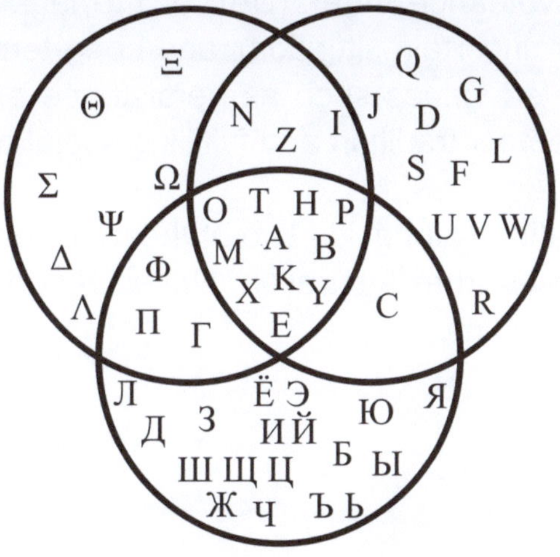

16. Which of the following conclusions **cannot** be supported by the Venn diagram?

A. The Greek alphabet does not share C with English and Russian.
B. Z is shared only by Greek and English alphabets.
C. Greek, Russian, and English alphabets share more vowels than consonants.
D. R is exclusively English.

17. Which pair of words can be made using the combination of Greek-English alphabets, but not the combination of Russian-English alphabets?

A. Home, path
B. Ozone, cable
C. Bait, biome
D. None of the above

Unit 6

Questions 18 - 20

Geert Hofstede is known for having empirically developed, with the help of IBM employees, a multidimensional model of cultural differences. Until the 2000s, it characterised nations along five main dimensions: Power Distance Index (PDI, or the acceptance that power is unequally distributed in organisations and that there are organisational hierarchies that must be respected); Individualism vs Collectivism (IND–COL, or the valuing of tight in-group social networks vs extended family networks); Masculinity vs Femininity (MAS-FEM, or the acceptance of the division of men and women's emotional roles, and the valuing of assertiveness, competitiveness, and material goods acquisition over quality of life and caring relationships); Uncertainty Avoidance Index (UAI, or the lack of tolerance and tendency to normalise and legislate every uncertain situation); and Long-term-Short-term orientation (LTO, or the holding of future-oriented values such as persistence and thrift vs past- and present-oriented values such as respect for tradition and fulfilling social obligations).

Figure 1 plots several nations alongside two of these dimensions, and Figure 2 shows the scores obtained with employees from Australian, United Kingdom (UK) and United States of America (USA) across five domains.

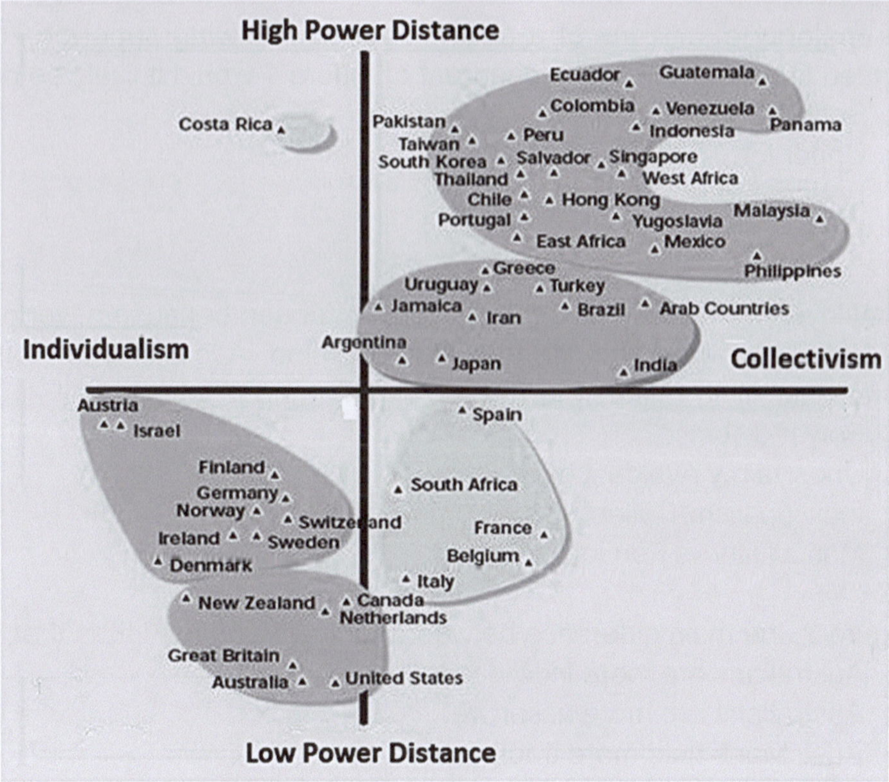

Figure 1. Worldwide nations along IND-COL and PDI dimensions.

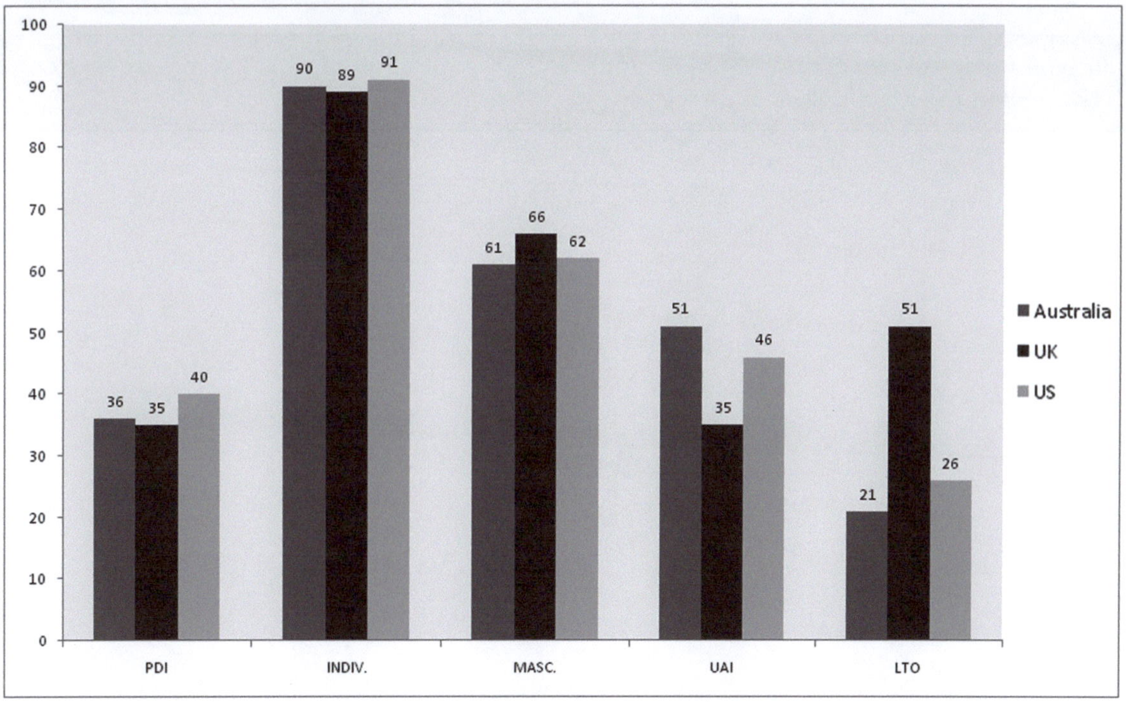

Figure 2. Australia scores over five Hofstede's dimensions.

Sources: G. Hofstede, G. J. Hofstede, & M. Minkov. "Cultures and Organizations, Software of the Mind", Third Revised Edition, McGrawHill Eds, ISBN 0-07-166418-1. Copyright 2010 Geert Hofstede B.V. Printed with permission.

18. If the majority of citizens of a nation disliked following superiors' orders and nurtured extended family ties, in which quadrant of Figure 1 would it likely be placed?

A. Bottom left
B. Upper left
C. Bottom right
D. Upper right

19. An employee from a different country feels offended because never once have colleagues asked about his personal life and state of mind. According to Hofstede's model, such cultural clash likely relates to which of the following dimensions?

A. Power distance
B. Uncertainty Avoidance
C. Individualism-Collectivism
D. Masculinity vs Femininity

20. In Figure 2, the main difference between Australia and the UK is that:

A. Australians are more individualist.
B. Australians are more assertive.
C. Australians hold more traditional values.
D. Australians are better able to deal with unstructured processes.

If time remains, you may re-examine your work. If your allotted time (32 minutes) is complete, please proceed to the Answer Key.

3.8.12 Graphs and Tables Test Answer Key and Worked Solutions

1. C	**5.** D	**9.** C	**13.** C	**17.** C
2. D	**6.** A	**10.** C	**14.** B	**18.** C
3. B	**7.** A	**11.** C	**15.** A	**19.** D
4. B	**8.** B	**12.** B	**16.** C	**20.** C

1. **Correct Answer: C**
As stated in the abstract objective: "to explore patients' approaches to the doctor's computer in the consultation and its influence on the patient–doctor relationship" this clearly confirms (C) as the correct answer.

2. **Correct Answer: D**
This question asks you to choose the LEAST correct option. The diagram demonstrates that (A) doctor-patient relationships are certainly influenced by the use of computers. The note and diagram explain that (B) hermeneutics are based on a mutual definition. The abstract results explain why (C) agrees with the meaning of hermeneutics.

The answer is (D). The use of a computer was part of the study's methodology and the doctor-patient interaction can be said to have been facilitated by a computer to a certain extent. However, this statement does not coincide with the concept of hermeneutics, which concerns the co-creation of meanings (i.e. the facilitation needs to be reciprocal).

3. **Correct Answer: B**
"Patients negotiated the relationship between themselves, the doctor, and the computer demonstrating two themes: dyadic (dealing primarily with the doctor) or triadic (dealing with both computor and doctor)." This quote from the results overview confirms (B) as the correct answer.

4. **Correct Answer: B**
The reference to Goffman's dramaturgy indicates (B) theatre as the correct answer: *"In this paper, the authors use Goffman's dramaturgy (theatrical approach: scene, actor, stage, script, act) to explore patients' approaches to the doctor's computer in the consultation and its influence on the patient–doctor relationship."*

5. **Correct Answer: D**
First, using a scratch pad, this would represent the corrected table - corrected scores are highlighted.

There are no errors in Claire's scores, indicating (D) as the correct answer.

	Judge's score *x*	**Score minus 8** *x-8*	**Tripled score** *3x*	**Cubed score** *x3*
Alice's cooking ability	10	2	30	1000
Bob's cooking ability	9	1	27	729
Claire's cooking ability	8.5	0.5	25.5	614.125
Dana's cooking ability	8	0	24	512
Edgar's cooking ability	5	-3	15	125

6. **Correct Answer: A**
The scores decrease steadily with Alice's scores to be the highest and Edgar's scores to be the lowest, indicating (A) as the correct answer. (B) Exponentially is incorrect because the decrease of scores would be in large quantitative amounts. (C) Parsimoniously is nonsense, while (D) regressively refers to best fit, smallest size decreases of numerical relations, more properly suited to statistical analysis techniques – this answer is a bit of a red herring or distraction. Also, the question stem already states that the scores are supposed to decrease (i.e. regress).

7. **Correct Answer: A**
To find the average, total the 5 scores and divide by 5. 30 + 27 + 25.5 + 24 + 15 = 121.5/5 = 24.3 This indicates (A) as the correct answer.

8. **Correct Answer: B**
First, find the average judge's score:
10 + 9 + 8.5 + 8 + 5 = 40.5
40.5/5 = 8.1 (Average Judge's Score)

To find the cubed score x3 (8.1 x 8.1 x 8.1). This results to 531.441 indicating (B) as the correct answer.

9. **Correct Answer: C**
A quick scan of the estimates and assumptions based on graphical data (33.65 bbl/d per citizen in the UK in 2000 and 23.35 bbl/d per citizen in Australia in 2000) indicates a rough difference of 10 bbl/d confirming (C) as the correct answer.

10. **Correct Answer: C**
Net imports refer to the difference between consumption and production. A trick for these kinds of questions is using a straight edge, like a ruler or piece of paper aligned across the graph. This alignment will roughly show the difference between 600,000 and 950,000 indicating (C) 350,000 bbl/d as the correct answer.

11. **Correct Answer: C**
A quick glance will affirm that (C) consumption has varied the least - making it the most consistent variable.

12. **Correct Answer: B**
(B) Phases 4 and 7 are central hubs of activity within the diagram connecting 3 and 5, as well as 6 and 7. The whole gist of the last paragraph, concerning the factors, stresses this importance in terms of behaviour change and its relation to health education strategies.

13. **Correct Answer: C**
This easy detail-oriented quick scan question is transparently (C).

14. **Correct Answer: B**
One can infer within the rubric of Health Promotion, of which both phases 5 and 6 are associated with. There is mutual dynamism occurring between "health education" and "policy regulation and organisation". The arrows are pointing to each other indicating a mutually defining, modifying or changing process. For these reasons, (B) mutual reciprocity is the correct answer. The other answers are incorrect because (A) linear orientation stresses a one-way, unidirectional flow of information. (C) applies to the arrows moving into phases 4 and 7, yet this does not address the internal relationship between 5 and 6 while (D) is simply irrelevant.

15. **Correct Answer: A**
Considering that the commentary and diagram are essentially concerned with health education in relation to behavioural change, (A) is the correct answer. The other answers are holistically related to the diagram itself but do not reflect the essential focus of behavioural change. Without these contextually defining factors, the diagram would be meaningless. The whole framework of the analysis is based on the factors as can be inferred from the commentary excerpt:

The PRECEDE-PROCEED framework is an approach to planning that examines the factors contributing to behaviour change*. . . These factors require that individuals be considered in the context of their community and social structures, and not in isolation, when planning communication or health education strategies.*

16. Correct Answer: C

A quick perusal of the Venn diagram will confirm that all propositions (A), (B), and (D) are true while (C) the correct answer cannot be supported by the Venn diagram.

17. Correct Answer: C

(A) HOME and PATH can be formed at both intersections.

(B) While OZONE can be formed in Greek-English alphabets, CABLE cannot be formed at either of the intersections.

(C) Only at the intersection of Greek-English alphabets can BAIT and BIOME be formed. This is because the letter "I" is exclusive at the Greek-English intersection. Of course, this makes option (D) wrong.

18. Correct Answer: C

The acceptance that power is unequally distributed and hierarchies must be respected are assessed via PDI. Those with low scores on this scale do not easily accept that their place in organisations is unquestionable and defined by their place within the organisational hierarchies. For a country with high PDI, this is understood as a lack of respect for superiors' orders. This would thus likely be associated with the bottom quadrants of Figure 1. The valuing and nurturing extended family ties, rather than the emotional bonds with a small set of individuals who may or may not belong to one's family, is associated with collectivism. This places the country to the right of Figure 1. Then, the nation should be placed on the bottom right side of the quadrant in Figure 1.

19. Correct Answer: D

The offended individual expected co-workers to establish an intimate, personal relationship with him/her. When colleagues failed to do so, they demonstrated how such line of querying and relating was not a cultural norm regulating their behaviour. That is, they clash in regards to the dimension MAS-FEM. This dimension taps into values such as the establishment of caring relationships (Femininity) vs the establishment of competitive, materialistic, and assertive relationships (Masculinity).

20. Correct Answer: C

According to Figure 2, the three nations are similar in terms of PDI, IND-COL, and MASC-FEM. They differ more in terms of UAI and LTO. Australians score slightly higher on UAI and lower on LTO. That is, they experience more of the need to regulate every interaction and procedure and thereby avoid the uncertainty of situations (UAI). They also, and more markedly, hold on to cultural/national traditions and mores.

High-level Importance

SPOILER ALERT

Gold Standard has cross-referenced the content in this chapter to examples from ACER's official GAMSAT practice materials. It is for you to decide when you want to explore these questions since you may want to preserve some of ACER's materials for timed mock-exam practice.

Examples – Graphs/Tables/Diagrams units Q7-12 of 2; Q23-25, Q49-52 and Q73-74 of 3; Q11-13, Q32-36, Q55-58 and Q59-64 of 4; Q6 and Q14 of 5. Note that "Q" is followed by the question number, and, for example, "of 1" refers to booklet number 1 which is referenced in the Spoiler Alert table at the end of section RHSS 3.2.4. The 15 full-length HEAPS GAMSAT practice tests (by Gold Standard) include exams that contain specific cross-references to this chapter within the worked solutions.

Chapter Checklist

- ☐ Access your online account to view answers, worked solutions and discussion boards.
- ☐ Complete a maximum of 1 page of notes using symbols/abbreviations to represent the content in the foregoing section. These are your Gold Notes.
- ☐ Consider your options based on your optimal way of learning:
  - ☐ Create your own, tangible study cards or try the free app: Anki.
  - ☐ Record your voice reading your Gold Notes onto your smartphone (MP3s) and listen during exercise, transportation, etc.
  - ☐ Consider reading at least 1 source material every day (e.g., poems of a single author, a synopsis of a novel, an article from a scientific journal that caught your interest, etc.). Note down the main idea or ideas of the piece on your scratch paper. Determine or surmise the author's sentiment or purpose for writing the material.
- ☐ Reassess your schedule for your full-length GAMSAT practice tests: ACER and/or HEAPS exams. Ensure that you have scheduled one full day to complete a practice test and 1-2 days for a thorough assessment of worked solutions while adding to your abbreviated Gold Notes.
- ☐ Reassess your progress in scheduling and/or evaluating stress reduction techniques such as regular exercise (sports), yoga, meditation and/or mindfulness exercises (*see* YouTube for suggestions).

CANDIDATE'S NAME ______________________________ BOOKLET GS1-I

STUDENT ID ______________________________

Note: This section of your Masters Series book contains 3 full-length Humanities and Social Sciences tests with the new digital-format GAMSAT timing. Only 1 test is from one of our 15 Gold Standard (GS)/HEAPS exams: GAMSAT Masters Series Test 1 comes from HEAPS-6 (AKA GS-1).

GAMSAT Masters Series Test 1

Reasoning in Humanities and Social Sciences

Questions: 1-62
Time: 100 minutes

INSTRUCTIONS: Of the 62 questions in this test, many are organised into groups preceded by stimulus material. After evaluating the stimulus material, select the best answer to each question in the group. Some questions are independent of any descriptive passage or each other. Similarly, select the best answer to these questions. If you are unsure of an answer, eliminate the alternatives that you know to be incorrect and select an answer from the remaining alternatives. To indicate your selection, use a pencil to circle the letter in your test booklet. If you wish to make notes, you may use two A4 sheets as scratch paper since this will be provided to you on test day for the new, digital GAMSAT (some test centres permit the use of whiteboards). No marks are deducted for wrong answers.

The Gold Standard GAMSAT* has been designed exclusively to test knowledge and thinking skills. The exam may contain hypothetical statements and/or express controversial ideas. Statements contained herein do not necessarily reflect the policy, position, or view of RuveneCo Inc.

OPEN BOOKLET ONLY WHEN TIMER IS READY.

Answers and worked solutions are available to the original owner at gamsat-prep.com.
(register at: www.gamsat-prep.com/gamsat-humanities-and-social-sciences)

UNIT 1

The following two passages discuss different indigenous values.

Questions 1 – 2 refer to Passage I.

PASSAGE I

"Mitakuye Oyasin" is a Native American prayer and expression. Even though it only consists of two words in the Lakota Sioux language, the expression is considered the most powerful prayer when uttered. The phrase translates roughly as "all my relations" and "we are all-connected", within the same utterance.

The Lakota Sioux also honoured, respected, and can be said to have worshipped the Buffalo. Their ceremonies had rites and rituals and every part of the animal, after it was killed, was used for food, clothing, tools, and weapons.

In many ways, the Lakota Sioux exhibited wisdom in their views of the environment. Their prayer implies that all life deserves honour and respect, because all life is valued, and intertwined with each other. Their rituals also showed that from the smallest ant to the greatest and strongest creatures of the Earth, all are connected and useful in a biological system.

1. For the Lakota Sioux, "honour and respect" connotes:
- **A** worship.
- **B** interconnection.
- **C** value.
- **D** parity.

2. ". . . all life deserves honour and respect, because all life is valued, and intertwined with each other" is closest to which Native American proverb?
- **A** Respect the gift and the giver.
- **B** When we show our respect for other living things, they respond with respect for us.
- **C** With all things and in all things, we are relatives.
- **D** Treat the earth well: it was not given to you by your parents; it was loaned to you by your children. We do not inherit the Earth from our Ancestors; we borrow it from our Children.

Questions 3 – 6 relate to either Passage II or both passages.

PASSAGE II

For the Indigenous Australians, kinship to the land is a core spiritual value. While geographical boundaries such as lakes, rivers, and mountains distinguish each Aboriginal clan, these "traditional lands" bind the identity of its people to their territory. There are areas in a territory that certain clan members have a special connection with, like for example, the place where one's mother first conceived. This gives them a deeper affinity, respect and care for that locale and the lives surrounding it.

Understandably, an Aboriginal clan does not only possess the right to use their land and benefit from its returns; they also take on the duty to cultivate and preserve their own environment, including its animals. As one Kakadu elders, Bill Neidjie puts it, "Our story is in the land. . . it is written in those sacred places. . . My Children will look after those places, that's the law."

3. The phrase "Our story is in the land" connotes that:
- **A** Aboriginal tribes are eternally bound to their land by tradition and history.
- **B** among the Aborigines in Australia, the land and identity are inseparable.
- **C** traditional lands embody the values and belief systems of the Aborigines.
- **D** Aboriginal folklore is rich in stories about the origins of their land.

4. According to the Indigenous Australians, "respect and care" for the environment is an expression of:
   A tribal worship.
   B ancestral affinity.
   C fiduciary duty.
   D ethnic custom.

5. The Lakota Sioux and the Aborigines of Australia are only two of the native tribes which were labelled by 17th century European colonisers as "savages". However, the indigenous values presented in the two passages parallel much of today's principles about ecology. Which of the following statements would alter the old European perception regarding the culture of these native people?
   A Indigenous people have always had a great sense of indebtedness and respect for the environment.
   B The culture of the natives has always been guided by natural insights as compared to the highbrow rationalism of the Europeans.
   C Native tribes have always had an advanced culture save for their unrefined wardrobe fashion.
   D Indigenous people have long had a sophisticated code of conduct, which includes the preservation of and the harmonious co-existence with nature.

6. In both passages, the following is a common idea on the environment:
   A both native cultures illustrate the interrelationships of all life.
   B both cultures honour and respect ecosystems.
   C indigenous tribes have a long history of worshipping nature.
   D the two passages highlight indigenous spiritual orientation.

UNIT 2

Questions 7 - 16

*The following is an excerpt from **The Grapes of Wrath** by John Steinbeck.*

The owners of the land came onto the land, or more often a spokesman for the owners came. They came in closed cars, and they felt the dry earth with their fingers, and sometimes they drove big earth augers into the ground for soil tests. The tenants, from their sun-beaten dooryards, watched uneasily when the closed cars drove along the fields. And at last the owner men drove into the dooryards and sat in their cars to talk out of the windows. The tenant men stood beside the cars for awhile, and then squatted on their hams and found sticks with which to mark the dust.

In the open doors the women stood looking out, and behind them the children – corn headed children, with wide eyes, one bare foot on top of the other bare foot, and the toes working. The women and the children watched their men talking to the owner men.

They were silent.

Some of the owner men were kind because they hated what they had to do, and some of them were angry because they hated to be cruel, and some of them were cold because they had long ago found that one could not be an owner unless one were cold. And all of them were caught in something larger than themselves. Some of them hated the mathematics that drove them, and some were afraid, and some worshipped the mathematics because it provided a refuge from thought and from feeling. If a bank or a finance company owned the land, the owner man said, The Bank – or the Company – needs – wants – insists – must have – as though the Bank or the Company were a monster, with thought and feeling, which had ensnared them. These last would take no responsibility for the banks or the companies because they were men and slaves, while the banks were machines and masters all at the same time. Some of the owner men were a little proud to be slaves to such cold and powerful masters.

The owner men sat in the cars and explained. "You know the land is poor. You've scrabbled at it long enough, God knows."

The squatting tenant men nodded and wondered and drew figures in the dust, and yes, they knew, God knows. If the dust only wouldn't fly. If the top would only stay on the soil, it might not be so bad.

The owner men went on leading to their point: "You know the land's getting poorer. You know what cotton does to the land; robs it, sucks all the blood out of it."

The squatters nodded – they knew, God knew. If they could only rotate the crops they might pump blood back into the land.

Well, it's too late. And the owner men explained the workings and the thinkings of the monster that was stronger than they were. "A man can hold land if he can just eat and pay taxes; he can do that."

"Yes, he can do that until his crops fail one day and he has to borrow money from the bank."

"But – you see, a bank or a company can't do that, because those creatures don't breathe air, don't eat side-meat. They breathe profits; they eat the interest on money. If they don't get it, they die the way you die without air, without side-meat. It is a sad thing, but it is so. It is just so."

7. The tenants are portrayed in the excerpt as:
- **A** hard workers.
- **B** poor and impoverished.
- **C** well rewarded.
- **D** lazy and incompetent.

8. "Monster" (line 17) in the passage refers to which of the following?
- **A** The Dust
- **B** The dying off of crops
- **C** The banking system
- **D** The owners of the land

9. The tone of the narrative in this passage suggests:
- **A** perseverance.
- **B** hopelessness.
- **C** rage.
- **D** anger.

10. The passage seems to describe a historical setting that took place during which American event listed below?
- **A** The Great Depression
- **B** World War 2
- **C** The Dust Bowl
- **D** The Great Immigration to the U.S.

11. "Scrabbled" (line 21) would mean:
- **A** squandered.
- **B** scrubbed away at.
- **C** squatted on.
- **D** tilled.

12. There are many references to "squatting" in the narrative. What would be the best definition listed below?
- **A** Waiting for good soil
- **B** Wasting time idly, not working
- **C** Staying on the land, to own it
- **D** Ready to get orders from the bosses

13. To some extent, the workers are portrayed as slaves in the excerpt. How are the bosses portrayed?
  A Mean, cruel, and without conscience
  B As slaves to the banks
  C Supportive of the worker's rights
  D As hard working farmers

14. Based on the excerpt, owners:
  A are genuinely concerned about the squatters.
  B are in cahoots with the banks.
  C want the squatters to leave.
  D have no interest in the squatters.

15. In this excerpt, the predominant image is:
  A machinery.
  B cotton.
  C soil.
  D dust.

16. In the colloquial phrase "cat side-meat" (lines 32-33), what does "cat" refer to?
  A Stealing
  B Eating
  C Hording
  D Portioning

Questions 17 – 18

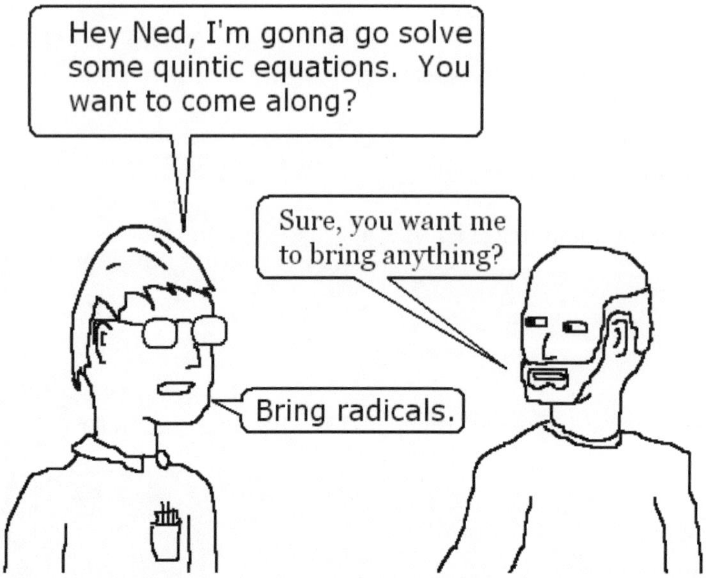

17. Even though we may not be familiar with quintic equations (which are polynomials as groups of 5, hence "quin"), the humour of this cartoon is due to which of the following?

A Maths and geeks
B The diversity of meanings in language
C The unintended irony
D The logical fallacies presented

18. We can infer from the party or social get together context of the cartoon that:

A there is always somebody radical at an event.
B radicals are very significant in relation to quintic equations.
C the get together is for brainiacs and maths whizzes.
D the author is not playing with language.

UNIT 4

Questions 19 – 21

The following is a short parable by the German philosopher Schopenhauer.

In a field of ripening corn I came to a place which had been trampled down by some ruthless foot; and as I glanced amongst the countless stalks, every one of them alike, standing there so erect and bearing the full weight of the ear, I saw a multitude of different flowers, red and blue and violet. How pretty they looked as they grew there so naturally with their little foliage! But, thought I, they are quite useless; they bear no fruit; they are mere weeds, suffered to remain only because there is no getting rid of them. And yet, but for these flowers, there would be nothing to charm the eye in that wilderness of stalks. They are emblematic of poetry and art, which, in civic life – so severe, but still useful and not without its fruit – play the same part as flowers in the corn.

19. The speaker in this parable regards the flowers as:
- **A** symbolic of the colours and abundance of life.
- **B** representative of the beautiful but useless in life.
- **C** unnecessary splendour that makes life bearable.
- **D** ideal symbols of poetic and artistic creations.

20. The parable suggests that the speaker regards poetry and art as:
- **A** superfluous.
- **B** purely ornamental.
- **C** uplifting.
- **D** purposive.

21. This parable could best be described as:
- **A** comparing and contrasting useful corn and beautiful flowers.
- **B** illustrating the functional aesthetics of poetry and art and nature.
- **C** pointing out how diverse nature is.
- **D** showing how poetry and flowers are like weeds.

UNIT 5

Questions 22 – 33

Extended Unit on Romanticism (in broken paragraphs)

PARAGRAPH I

The Romantic era, period, or movement, can be viewed as an artistic, political, and philosophical response to classical ideals and political dogma, the burgeoning paradigm of scientific rationalism, and the emergence of the industrial revolution. Within the historical context of the French and American Revolution, the individual was gaining new liberties over tyranny. The romantic hero emerged as a cultural icon becoming manifested in literary, philosophical, and historical stereotypes.

22. In Paragraph I, why would scientific rationalism, be considered a burgeoning paradigm?

A Because as a model of inquiry, it would be the dominant example to follow.
B Because the experimental method was beginning.
C Because technological innovations were at the forefront of culture.
D Because it was in direct opposition to poetic modes of thought.

PARAGRAPH II

Emphasising subjective experience over objective agreement, as in Browning's phrase "the mind is a thousand times more beautiful than nature could ever be", the romantic hero became a common figure in lyrical poetry and theatre. This passionate, talented hero, rejects societal ideals and norms, yet is instilled with some tragic flaw, which leads to his demise. Imbued with the attainment of perfection, the romantic hero could easily utter Browning's remarks, "A man's reach must exceed his grasp, or what is a heaven for?"

23. In reference to one of Lord Byron's major works, he is often quoted as saying: "Man's greatest tragedy is that he can conceive of a perfection which he cannot attain." Lord Byron's statement and Browning's "A man's reach must exceed his grasp, or what is a heaven for":

A differ in their perceptions of a perfect society.
B differ in their outlook towards man's pursuit of achieving perfection.
C are similar in their positive views about obtaining a perfect world.
D are similar in their assumptions about the nature of worldly pursuits.

PARAGRAPH III

Such is the basic nature of Moliere and Lord Byron's "Don Juan", whose unattainable appetites and libertine excesses bring about his own downfall. During this era, William Blake, visionary poet, remarked "the road of excess leads to the palace of wisdom" as if predefining a Byronic type of hero. Byron's own exploits paralleled his literary creations, as well, as a kind of "unattainable excess". Keats would describe this affliction or obsession as "egotistical sublime", and we find it in different personae in this era. Goethe's Faust suffers from the same malady but also ultimately redeems himself.

24. Paragraph III implies that, for Keats, a typical Byronic hero:

A is a failed perfectionist.
B is an obsessive, soul-searching hero.
C has no defined identity.
D is an excessive pleasure-seeker.

PARAGRAPH IV

In history, we find this same overachieving ego-figure in Napoleon, releasing the serfs from oppression, insisting on equality, founding the Napoleonic code of law, extending his megalomaniacal military reaches across the globe, until he is turned away from Russia, and defeated at Waterloo. Finally Napoleon was exiled, like The Count of Monte Cristo, and brought down by his own lust for power.

25. When describing Napoleon's military reaches, the term "megalomaniacal" is used. This term roughly equates to:
A slovenliness.
B prestige.
C military-like.
D ego.

PARAGRAPH V

The maestro violinist, Niccolò Paganini, whose persecution by the Church, can be seen as a romantic hero. Undeterred in his efforts to compose and perform, many legends and myths surround him. Supposedly slowly poisoned by mercury used to treat his tertiary syphilis, he was believed to be a fiddling devil, being able to play virtuoso on one string, caricatured as the mad genius who sold his soul, much like Faust. Being that the romantic mind was fascinated with things distorted or beyond nature, in a word – grotesque, as evidenced in Mary Shelley's Frankenstein, the demonic character of Paganini was a perfect example of how romantic ideas could enter into popular folklore.

26. In Paragraph V, the association between a romantic mind and the characters of Frankenstein and Paganini suggests that:
A being experimental was a Romantic tendency.
B the Romantic Movement was preoccupied with the unconventional and bizarre.
C the duality of human nature polarised between the sinister and the extraordinary, between good and evil, was a typical characteristic of a Romantic hero.
D Romanticism was distorted.

PARAGRAPH VI

While the beginnings of the scientific method were being refined, many poets and philosophers stood in bleak contrast to the rational logico-deductive models, and also drifted away from the classical Apollonian muses. In fact, the concept of imagination was offered by the romantics as diametrically opposed. "We murder to dissect" was Wordsworth's herald and "contemplation of nature" was given the highest priority against reductionist forms of thought. By finding voice in Dionysian modes of expression, without the Hellenic order and restraint of tempered metre or rhyme, these romantics located truth in the individual. In philosophy, subjective idealism was finding its groundings in Leibniz and Berkeley, and later more radically, with Nietzsche. In Germany, the romantic virtuoso was Beethoven and later Wagner, whose operas portrayed the pinnacle of German Romanticism, with its excessive exuberance, reigniting Nordic myths into national epics.

27. Wordsworth's quote in Paragraph IV, "We murder to dissect" is a poetic response to:
A extreme egoism.
B the fatal flaw.
C fallacies of myth.
D the scientific method.

28. In Paragraph VI, an opposition between the classical Greek gods – Apollo and Dionysus – symbolises which of the following?
A Truth and Illusion
B Order and Freedom
C Music and Poetry
D Ego and Pride

PARAGRAPH VII

Blake, Wordsworth, Keats, Shelley, et al. helped define poets "as unacknowledged legislators of the world, (Shelley)," who should break free of "the mind-forged manacles (Blake)" of contemporary thought through contemplation with and of nature. Keats' "Truth is Beauty, Beauty is Truth" is symptomatic of the romantic impulse to find an alternative to the reductive process of science, which many poets found "dissective" in its scope and process.

Perhaps the epitome and end of Romantic philosophers can be found in Nietzsche, who in virtual isolation from humanity, writes of a greater humanity, located in the 'Superman', beyond good and evil. Peering into the abyss and limits of philosophy, as such, brought about his own downfall in the form of madness.

29. According to Paragraph VII, which of the following is NOT true about the Romantic era?
- **A** The Romantic era was concerned with individual experience.
- **B** The Romantic era sought freedom from different constraints.
- **C** The Romantic era was concerned with contemplation with Nature.
- **D** The Romantic era was logical and scientific.

30. The description of Nietzsche "who in virtual isolation from humanity, writes of a greater humanity" is an example of what?
- **A** Madness
- **B** Contradiction
- **C** Irony
- **D** Metaphor

Questions 31 – 33 pertain to all paragraphs.

31. Which of the following statements does NOT describe the Romantic spirit implied in the preceding paragraphs?
- **A** Do what you will, this world's a fiction and is made up of contradiction.
- **B** Come forth into the light of things, let nature be your teacher.
- **C** I have love in me the likes of which you can scarcely imagine. A rage, the likes of which you would not believe. If I cannot satisfy one, I will indulge in the other.
- **D** I love you the more in that I believe you had liked me for my own sake and for nothing else.

32. A certain type of support in relation to the author's interpretation was extensively used in the paragraphs. Which of the following would be the best answer in defining this type of support?
- **A** Historical examples
- **B** Literary quotations
- **C** Various juxtapositions
- **D** Contrasting analogies

33. Based on the paragraphs, the term "subjective" in the Romantic context is:
- **A** outside, verifiable.
- **B** dependent upon.
- **C** subject to.
- **D** personal, individual.

Questions 34 – 37

The following is Graham's "Hierarchy of Disagreement".

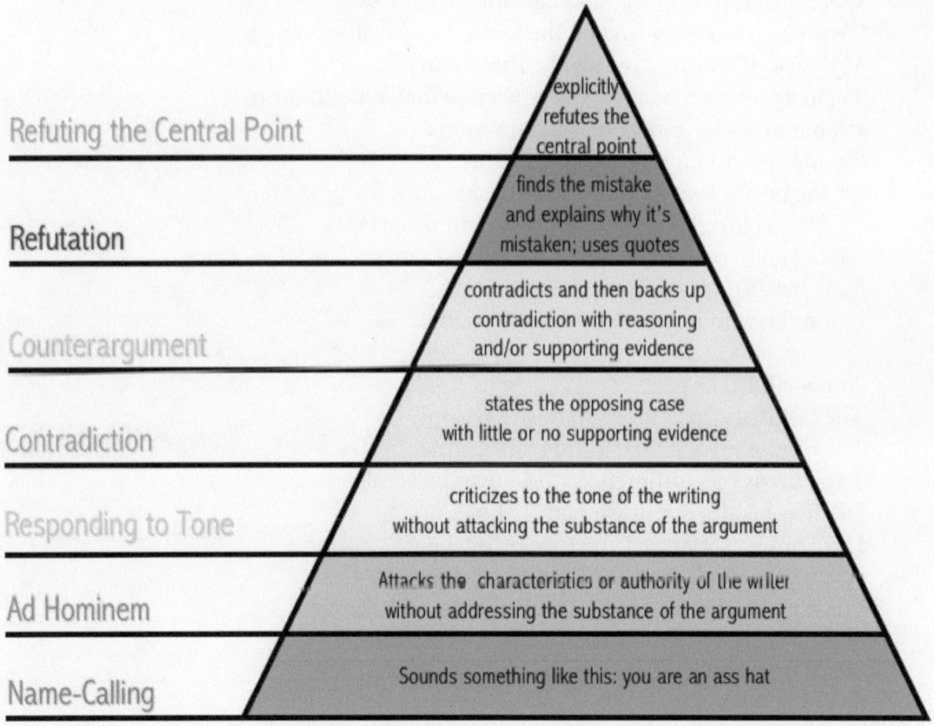

34. Based on the diagram, what makes "Responding to Tone" a weak form of disagreement?
- **A** Tone is hard to judge.
- **B** It overlooks the correctness of the writer's point.
- **C** The response is still fundamentally a personal attack on the writer.
- **D** It allows the critic to disagree without valid evidence.

35. This diagram shows that:
- **A** it is necessary to differentiate between name-calling and Ad Hominem attacks.
- **B** refuting the main point of an argument does not need supporting evidence.
- **C** the tone of the argument is more important than the substance of the argument.
- **D** the hierarchy moves from an emotional response to logical refutation.

36. Graham's "Hierarchy of Disagreement" seems to emphasise that:
- **A** argumentation is inherently impassioned.
- **B** anger makes argumentation personal.
- **C** disagreeing essentially means arguing.
- **D** it is possible to disagree without necessarily being angry.

37. The disagreement hierarchy is presented in the form of a pyramid in order to show that:
- **A** disagreements occur in stages.
- **B** forms of disagreement are arranged in an ascending manner.
- **C** the more rational the disagreement, the less it is employed.
- **D** rationality should govern disagreements.

Questions 38 – 42

Afternoon in School - The Last Lesson

When will the bell ring, and end this weariness?
How long have they tugged the leash, and strained apart
My pack of unruly hounds: I cannot start
Them again on a quarry of knowledge they hate to hunt,
I can haul them and urge them no more.
No more can I endure to bear the brunt
Of the books that lie out on the desks: a full three score
Of several insults of blotted pages and scrawl
Of slovenly work that they have offered me.
I am sick, and tired more than any thrall
Upon the woodstacks working weariedly.

And shall I take
The last dear fuel and heap it on my soul
Till I rouse my will like a fire to consume
Their dross of indifference, and burn the scroll
Of their insults in punishment? - I will not!
I will not waste myself to embers for them,
Not all for them shall the fires of my life be hot,
For myself a heap of ashes of weariness, till sleep
Shall have raked the embers clear: I will keep
Some of my strength for myself, for if I should sell
It all for them, I should hate them -
- I will sit and wait for the bell.

D. H. Lawrence

38. The learning atmosphere depicted in the poem is:
A exhausting because of the healthy exchange of ideas.
B challenging.
C unruly and hateful.
D indifferent, therefore pointless.

39. What is meant by "slovenly work" (line 9)?
A Done obediently like a dog
B Repetitive and unnecessary
C Terse and unfocused
D Done in a hasty and sloppy fashion

40. The literary style of Lawrence's poem, with its series of rhetorical questions, theatrically most resembles a(n):
A dialogue.
B soliloquy.
C imbrications.
D aside.

41. Line 23 suggests that the attitude of the speaker is one of:
A impatience.
B detachment.
C resignation.
D frustration.

42. The ringing of the bell in this poem connotes:

A a relief from boredom.
B freedom from the burdens of teaching.
C a signal of opportunity for the speaker to channel his noble efforts to a more rewarding endeavour.
D hope for a better classroom situation the next day.

UNIT 8

Questions 43 – 47

From late 1950s to early 1960s, the issue of African-American Civil Rights was crucial in shaping the eventual structure of politics and image of democracy in America. The following are excerpts from speeches of two of the most influential advocate-leaders of the time.

Questions 43 – 44 pertain to Passage I.

PASSAGE I

The political philosophy of black nationalism means that the black man should control the politics and the politicians in his own community; no more. The black man in the black community has to be re-educated into the science of politics so he will know what politics is supposed to bring him in return. Don't be throwing out any ballots. A ballot is like a bullet. You don't throw your ballots until you see a target, and if that target is not within your reach, keep your ballot in your pocket.

The political philosophy of black nationalism is being taught in the Christian church. It's being taught in the NAACP. It's being taught in CORE meetings. It's being taught in SNCC Student Nonviolent Coordinating Committee meetings. It's being taught in Muslim meetings. It's being taught where nothing but atheists and agnostics come together. It's being taught everywhere.

Black people are fed up with the dillydallying, pussyfooting, compromising approach that we've been using toward getting our freedom. We want freedom now, but we're not going to get it saying "We Shall Overcome." We've got to fight until we overcome.

The economic philosophy of black nationalism is pure and simple. It only means that we should control the economy of our community. Why should white people be running all the stores in our community? Why should white people be running the banks of our community? Why should the economy of our community be in the hands of the white man? Why? If a black man can't move his store into a white community, you tell me why a white man should move his store into a black community. The philosophy of black nationalism involves a re-education program in the black community in regards to economics. Our people have to be made to see that any time you take your dollar out of your community and spend it in a community where you don't live, the community where you live will get poorer and poorer, and the community where you spend your money will get richer and richer.

"The Ballot or the Bullet" by Malcolm X
(Founder, Muslim Mosque Inc.)
April 3 1964

43. Based on the passage, Malcolm X associates the ballot with:

A wise decision-making.
B freedom to act out one's choice.
C a means for achieving advancement.
D civil rights.

44. Malcolm X proposes that the way for African-Americans to attain freedom is through:
- **A** a drastic change in the national political system.
- **B** the indoctrination of Black Nationalism.
- **C** exigent measures.
- **D** voting wisely.

PASSAGE II

Every American citizen must have an equal right to vote.

There is no reason which can excuse the denial of that right. There is no duty which weighs more heavily on us than the duty we have to ensure that right.

Yet the harsh fact is that in many places in this country men and women are kept from voting simply because they are Negroes. Every device of which human ingenuity is capable has been used to deny this right. The Negro citizen may go to register only to be told that the day is wrong, or the hour is late, or the official in charge is absent. And if he persists, and if he manages to present himself to the registrar, he may be disqualified because he did not spell out his middle name or because he abbreviated a word on the application. And if he manages to fill out an application, he is given a test. The registrar is the sole judge of whether he passes this test.

He may be asked to recite the entire Constitution, or explain the most complex provisions of State law. And even a college degree cannot be used to prove that he can read and write.

For the fact is that the only way to pass these barriers is to show a white skin. Experience has clearly shown that the existing process of law cannot overcome systematic and ingenious discrimination. No law that we now have on the books – and I have helped to put three of them there – can ensure the right to vote when local officials are determined to deny it. In such a case our duty must be clear to all of us. The Constitution says that no person shall be kept from voting because of his race or his colour. We have all sworn an oath before God to support and to defend that Constitution. We must now act in obedience to that oath.

from "We Shall Overcome" by Lyndon Baines Johnson
(Thirteenth President of the United States)
March 16 1965

Questions 45 – 47 apply to either Passage II or both passages.

45. Former U.S. President Johnson views equality in voting rights as a(n):
- **A** social responsibility.
- **B** constitutional right.
- **C** political duty.
- **D** affirmation of freedom.

46. In reference to the failure of granting equal rights to the African-Americans, both speakers assign the culpability to:
- **A** the biased government system.
- **B** segregation.
- **C** cunning politicians.
- **D** arbitrary legal provisions.

47. The two passages seem to suggest that:
- **A** Malcolm X favours racial segregation while President Johnson favours integration.
- **B** unlike Malcolm X, President Johnson maintains his confidence in the U.S. Constitution.
- **C** both speakers claim that the government is responsible for racial inequities in America.
- **D** Malcolm X views the act of voting as a choice while President Johnson views it as a must.

Questions 48 – 49

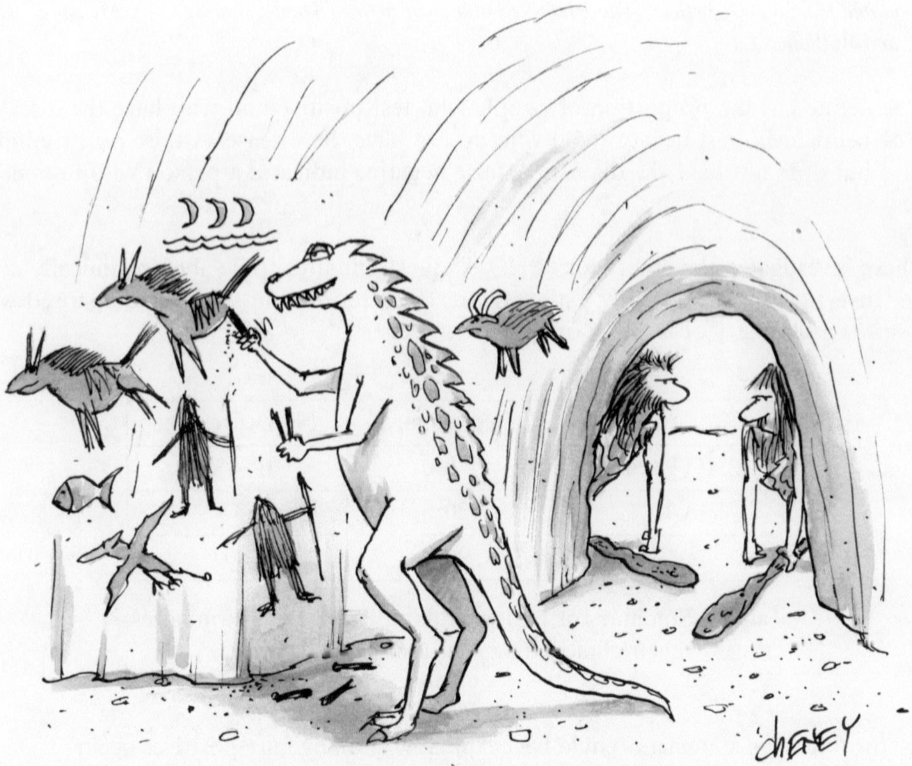

"It will be worth even more when he's extinct."

Used with permission. Credit: Tom Cheney/The New Yorker Collection/The Cartoon Bank

48. Which of the following attitudes towards art in society is suggested by this image?
- **A** Art only has meaning once the artist is dead.
- **B** The art one makes before they are famous is worth more than the art made after.
- **C** Only with retrospect can we appreciate an artist's work.
- **D** The value of one's art is arbitrary until there is a finite number of artworks.

49. The tone of this image and its caption is:
- **A** reverent.
- **B** cynical.
- **C** hopeful.
- **D** sardonic.

Questions 50 – 51

The following is adapted from a 2001 article "The PHQ-9: Validity of a Brief Depression Severity Measure" written by Kroenke, K., Spitzer, R. L., and Williams, J. B.

Sensitivity can be defined as the proportion of people who test positive and who have the disease. Specificity is the proportion of people who test negative and who do not have the disease. A false positive indicates a person who tests positive but does not have the disease. A false negative indicates a person who tests negative but does have the disease.

Recent studies have investigated the ability for "PHQ-9" questionnaires to be able to clinically diagnose patients with depression. Investigators set that any patient score 10 or more points will be diagnosed with depression. Table 1, below, shows a summary of a subset of data.

	Depression	**No Depression**
PHQ 9 score	n=110	n=475
< 10	20	415
>=10	90	60

Table 1 Summary of patients taking PHQ-9 questionnaires, their clinical diagnosis and PHQ-9 score.

50. Which of the following statements could best explain why many false positives occur?

A People tend to overplay the extent of their answers when tested.
B Young adolescent women were over represented in the number of people questioned.
C Men usually hide their emotions.
D The questionnaire is not a useful tool for assessing whether a person is depressed

51. A psychiatric society has deemed a mental health test accurate if it has a sensitivity of greater than 80%.

Given the information provided what can be said regarding the study?

I. Comparisons cannot be made between the two populations due to the large difference in sizes.
II. This test will be suitable for the needs of the psychiatric society.
III. 30% of the population is likely to be depressed.

A I only
B II only
C I and II only
D I, II, and III

Questions 52 – 56

The following commentaries were extracted from a 2011 article written by Huddle, T. S., & Maletz, K. K. L. (2011): "Physician Involvement with Politics—Obligation or Avocation?"

Dr. Mills and Dr. Ribeira are having a conversation in the hospital break room. Dr. Mills is complaining about another physician, Dr. George, because Dr. George is heavily involved in lobbying his local congressman for patient-centered health reform.

"He'd be doing a lot more good," Dr. Mills suggests, "if he spent less time following politics and more time reading medical journals. In my opinion, the best way for physicians to provide quality care for their patients is to be competent, careful, compassionate, and spend their extra time learning about the latest treatment recommendations. Not only that," he adds, "George is so wrapped up in partisan politics, writing and arguing with his congressman. I don't see how he can remain unbiased and patient-centered in his practice."

Dr. Ribeira disagrees and, in fact, applauds Dr. George's patient advocacy, noting that if physicians don't contribute to an informed discussion of health reform, from whom should legislators obtain information? He expresses a belief that physicians have a duty to advocate for sound health policy. "The Dr. Marcus Welby days are over, my friend," he says to Dr. Mills. "We have a simple choice today: work to enact policy that will help medicine or have someone else force politically motivated regulations on us."

52. What best describes Dr George's behaviour according to Dr Mills (lines 9-11)?
- **A** Dismissive
- **B** Sanctimonious
- **C** Pre-occupied
- **D** Obssessed

53. What statement most accurately reflects opinions Dr Marcus Welby might share?
- **A** The physician must be compassionate, well-informed, and be a strong advocate for patients.
- **B** My strongest asset is my kind bedside manner; it is important to be on a first name basis with all my patients.
- **C** Understanding mechanisms and research behind medications and their efficacy trials is as important as inciting change to health law.
- **D** The doctors' role is limited to facilitating treatment in a competent, careful, and compassionate manner.

Questions 54 – 56 are preceded by commentaries provided by practicing doctors.

Commentary I

by Thomas S. Huddle, MD, PhD

Dr. Mills finds fault with a colleague, and Dr. Ribeira defends him. As is perhaps typical of conversations in hospital break rooms, each is more concerned with expressing an opinion than with carefully articulating and defending a position. Dr. Mills is overly impatient with Dr. George. Dr. George's preoccupation with politics need not imply that he neglects the medical literature. Nor does his involvement with politics signify an improper influence affecting his medical practice. Many physicians pursue more or less absorbing avocations alongside professional work, and their professional work is unimpeded. Dr. Mills has offered no particular grounds for supposing that politics is interfering with Dr. George's practice. Medicine need not, and, likely, ought not to occupy the whole of any physician's life. Politics is but one of many possible avocations, but there is no reason to think that it is especially incompatible with medicine.

54. What statement best summarises the author's views?
- **A** Doctors are highly opinionated and rarely listen to others.
- **B** Doctors are able to multi-task patient care and politics while working.
- **C** It is likely that physicians have opinions and interests outside of medicine.
- **D** It is likely that physicians are able to balance their work-life and other interests without the two interfering with one another.

Commentary II

by Kristina L. Maletz, MD

As this case shows, physicians today garner both respect and suspicion when involved in political affairs. A Gallup poll during the height of the health care reform debate showed a high degree of trust in physician involvement. Overall, the poll showed greater public trust in physicians' ideas for reform than in those of health care academicians, politicians, or commercial groups. Almost three-quarters of Americans expressed confidence in physicians to do the right thing in changing the health care delivery system; only half as many felt that way about congressional leaders.

55. The poll (lines 4-5) showed that greater public is more likely to trust ideas of physicians compared to those of health care academics. Why might this be the case?
- **A** Doctors are generally thought to be intelligent and hard workers.
- **B** Doctors are responsible for patient care.
- **C** Doctors are knowledgeable in healthcare law.
- **D** Doctors are more likely to understand the needs for patients.

56. What statement best reflects views that the authors of commentaries I and II would share?
- **A** Physicians are capable of coercing change in the healthcare system independently.
- **B** Physicians should assist in enacting change in the healthcare system.
- **C** The best physicians are those that focus on the quality of care for their patients.
- **D** Physicians should be encouraged to enter partisan political debates with colleagues and patients.

UNIT 12

Questions 57 – 62

The following is adapted from an article written by Shu-Ju Ada Cheng, which was published in the International and Multidisciplinary Journal of Social Sciences in 2013.

In the past two decades, there has been an increasing trend among researchers in social sciences of using mixed methods. Supporters point out that mixed methods can provide different answers to our inquiry. They argue that, to understand the larger-scale social pattern and the question of 'what', the quantitative method would be most effective. The qualitative method, confined to limited localities and subjects, can be used to understand the subjectivity of actors and questions of 'why' and 'how'. Supporters further point out that, since quantitative data is generalisable while qualitative data is not, these two methods are complementary.

Combining these two methods can generate the most comprehensive results. The trend toward combining both methods seems to derive from feminist scholars' critiques of quantitative methods, positivism, and scientific paradigms since the second wave women's movement. They point out that science is not neutral. It emerges under particular historical, social, and cultural contexts. Science is embedded with gender, racial, and cultural ideologies. Racial minority scholars have also made similar arguments, examining how science is developed under the context of racism and imperialism during the 19th century.

Social scientists are located within particular social and cultural contexts. Feminist scholars point out that social research treats male as the universal subject and generalises men's experiences to women. This epistemological and methodological bias ignores women's experiences. Since the 1970s, feminist scholars have focused on women, mostly using qualitative methods. While qualitative research has gained recognition and changed the methodological landscape in sociology over the past three decades, qualitative methods are still deemed less prestigious, rigorous, objective, and scientific. Criticisms include that it is too subjective, not rigorous enough, and not objective enough. It lacks generalisability and representativeness.

This disciplinary emphasis on the legitimacy of quantitative methods influences not only junior and or senior sociologists' methodological choices but also master and doctoral students' preferences. For students who are in the job market, quantitative skills meet the market demand. With the disciplinary emphasis and job market demands, students tend to choose quantitative methods as the main skill they would like to pursue. Further, with the pressure of tenure, junior scholars might also use quantitative research to claim the legitimacy of their research.

This institutional emphasis on quantitative research dictates a less recognised position of qualitative methods in social sciences disciplines. For many sociology programmes, at least in my programme, there are two levels of graduate courses on methodology. First level is an introductory course on general social science research methods. The second level is a qualitative methods course and several quantitative methods courses, such as advanced statistics, data analysis, and regression, etc. The teaching of introductory courses and the choice of textbooks further solidify the position of quantitative methods. Most introductory textbooks are usually written from the quantitative orientation and positivistic paradigm. Therefore, students are exposed to an epistemology and methodology rooted in positivism, with specific language, discourse, and lenses. Students are taught to think in terms of variables, hypothesis, objectivity, generalisability, and representativeness. They are taught to master tools rather than understanding their epistemological foundations.

The institutionalisation of quantification and the standardisation of curriculum make it difficult for me to teach qualitative methods. Students come to class expecting to learn skills as opposed to the intellectual and epistemological foundation of both methods. I start my class with critiquing scientific paradigm and positivism and presenting various paradigms in social science research. I want to emphasise that all research methods are value-laden. I discuss the historical, structural, and cultural contexts within which quantitative methods become dominant in American sociology, such as the establishment of foundations and funding agencies as well as the bureaucratisation of government agencies. Second, I want students to think of methods as contextualised and historicised. I bring out issues that are central to feminist scholarship, e.g., the unequal power relationship between the researcher and the research subject, the influence of the social location and identity of the researcher, subjectivity, reflexivity, exploitation, voices of subjects, and researcher's authority in interpretation and writing.

57. What is the author's main purpose for writing this passage?

A To argue that qualitative methods are just as important as quantitative, and that undervaluing them has negative consequences.
B To trace the history of qualitative sociological methods in the context of feminism and race studies.
C To weigh the pluses and minuses of including qualitative methods in sociological curriculums.
D To critique the use of quantitative methods in sociology as a practice that can reinforce existing power structures.

58. Lines 5 - 7 imply which of the following about qualitative research?

A Its methods are the same no matter what the topic or who the researcher is.
B It is suited to different topics and populations than quantitative research is.
C It is most commonly used in mixed research combined with quantitative research.
D It produces detailed information about a relatively small population or group of people.

59. Feminist scholarship, according to the passage:

A rejects qualitative research as patriarchal.
B is not as value-laden as traditional research.
C aims to give equal power to researchers and their subjects.
D aims to give equal attention to men's and women's experiences.

60. Which of the following could not be considered a good use of qualitative research methods?

- **A** A study on black women who are the first in their families to attend college exploring how they cope with the stress of the new environment
- **B** A study on small family farmers in northern Nebraska attempting to explain why some choose to sell their farms and others do not
- **C** A study on a small group of gay Republicans describing the stresses their identities and party affiliation place on them
- **D** A study on prescription painkiller addicts across the U.S. attempting to discover how many succeed in obtaining the drugs through legal means.

61. Which of the following potential discoveries would best support the author's claim that "science is not neutral"?

- **A** When surveyed about their levels of happiness, women report higher levels than men relative to their actual happiness because they have been conditioned to express themselves positively.
- **B** A meta-analysis showed that among studies claiming to have found a statistically significant result, 27% of the results could actually have been the result of random chance.
- **C** Most psychological studies use college students as subjects, but since U.S. college students are 60% female, the makeup of the studies does not accurately reflect that of the population.
- **D** A study on confirmation bias was published in a prestigious journal, but upon further review, it was found that the article misreported statistical findings, and it was retracted.

62. Lines 31 - 36 argue that the disciplinary emphasis on quantitative research shapes students' career choices. This discussion implies which of the following about professional development?

- **A** A graduate student's choice of what to study should be free from outside influence.
- **B** Graduate students should be encouraged to give equal weight to quantitative and qualitative methods.
- **C** Market forces dissuade students from studying research methods that might otherwise interest them.
- **D** Students may regret their choice not to study qualitative research and will be unable to learn them later in their careers.

CANDIDATE'S NAME ______________________________ BOOKLET GS1-II

STUDENT ID ______________________________

GAMSAT Masters Series Test 2

Reasoning in Humanities and Social Sciences

Questions: 1-62
Time: 100 minutes

INSTRUCTIONS: Of the 62 questions in this test, many are organised into groups preceded by stimulus material. After evaluating the stimulus material, select the best answer to each question in the group. Some questions are independent of any descriptive passage or each other. Similarly, select the best answer to these questions. If you are unsure of an answer, eliminate the alternatives that you know to be incorrect and select an answer from the remaining alternatives. To indicate your selection, use a pencil to circle the letter in your test booklet. If you wish to make notes, you may use two A4 sheets as scratch paper since this will be provided to you on test day for the new, digital GAMSAT (some test centres permit the use of whiteboards). No marks are deducted for wrong answers.

The Gold Standard GAMSAT* has been designed exclusively to test knowledge and thinking skills. The exam may contain hypothetical statements and/or express controversial ideas. Statements contained herein do not necessarily reflect the policy, position, or view of RuveneCo Inc.

OPEN BOOKLET ONLY WHEN TIMER IS READY.

Answers and worked solutions are available to the original owner at gamsat-prep.com.
(register at: www.gamsat-prep.com/gamsat-humanities-and-social-sciences)

UNIT 1

Questions 1 – 3

The following excerpt is from a 2015 article "Voices and the imaginative ear" written by Peter Garratt in ***The Lancet.***

Hear the voice of the bard,
Who present, past and future sees,
Whose ears have heard
The Holy Word,
That walked among the ancient trees

Blake's opening to the introductory poem of his Songs of Innocence and Experience (1794) discloses a model of poetry based upon voice-hearing: whoever is called to the occasion of the poet's words must take up a relation to a speaking voice, they insist, a voice invested with mystical authority (the Bard of oral tradition, inspired and prophetic). This command-like voice speaks of itself and its own creative necessity. But the lines also reveal Blake's bard to be first an auditor, a listener who becomes a voice, "Whose ears have heard / The Holy Word". The poet harnesses the power of speech from some primary ability to hear. From the start, his voice mingles with a greater originating power. Blake is extending a long tradition of associating literary inspiration with the accommodation of strange voices, a view stretching from Plato's theory of divine madness to the Romantic period's discovery of the creative imagination and beyond. To be inspired means giving oneself over to compelling forces at the fringes of being.

In a poetic fragment by William Wordsworth, the poet describes hearing the river Derwent as a voice of inspiration:

Standing beneath these elms, I hear thy voice,
Beloved Derwent, that peculiar voice
Heard in the stillness of the evening air,
Half-heard and half-created.

What, and where, is the "voice" of Wordsworth's river? Its noise occurs outside and inside the head, conjured in some strange act of hearing in which world and mind collaborate and conspire. Its "peculiar voice" is not so much out there, wholly alien, as already known, distinctive, joined to memory. We're assured of the poet's physical presence and yet the lines suggest that the Derwent's burbling is, in part, internally derived. And as the river's voice merges into, or emerges as, the verbal performance of the poem, it becomes difficult to tell apart his acts of hearing, remembering, imagining, and writing. But, again, what is this voice? At once, it is and isn't Wordsworth's voice. It could be that he hears his own creative inner speech somehow afresh, reinvigorated, in the sound of rushing water, since it offers an acoustic context happily conducive to poetry. Or is it that in the poet's ear some less easily identified voice makes itself heard?

1. Blake's bard is described as 'a listener who becomes a voice' (lines 11 - 13). In the first poem, what is the relationship between the listener and the voice?

A The listener is a prophet, relaying the voice of a higher power.
B The listener and the voice are one divine being.
C The listener accommodates the voices of nature.
D The listener is a vessel for the voice of a divine power.

2. Which of the following phrases best exemplifies Plato's theory of divine madness (lines 15 - 18) as referred to by the author?

A Inspiration is a period of manic religious hysteria.
B Madness is a gift of inspiration from God.
C Creativity is only accessible from an unstable mind.
D The gods are illogical, incongruous, and often unreasonable.

3. In comparison with the voice in Blake's poem, Wordsworth's voice is:

A less material.
B less spiritual.
C more disconcerting.
D more removed.

UNIT 2

Questions 4 – 7

*The following passage is an excerpt from the book, **Memoirs of Extraordinary Popular Delusions and the Madness of Crowds**, written by Scottish journalist Charles Mackay.*

Some in clandestine companies combine;
Erect new stocks to trade beyond the line;
With air and empty names beguile the town,
And raise new credits first, then cry 'em down;
Divide the empty nothing into shares,
And set the crowd together by the ears.--Defoe.

The personal character and career of one man are so intimately connected with the great scheme of the years 1719 and 1720, that a history of the Mississippi madness can have no fitter introduction than a sketch of the life of its great author John Law. Historians are divided in opinion as to whether they should designate him a knave or a madman. Both epithets were unsparingly applied to him in his lifetime, and while the unhappy consequences of his projects were still deeply felt. Posterity, however, has found reason to doubt the justice of the accusation, and to confess that John Law was neither knave nor madman, but one more deceived than deceiving, more sinned against than sinning. He was thoroughly acquainted with the philosophy and true principles of credit. He understood the monetary question better than any man of his day; and if his system fell with a crash so tremendous, it was not so much his fault as that of the people amongst whom he had erected it.

He did not calculate upon the avaricious frenzy of a whole nation; he did not see that confidence, like mistrust, could be increased almost *ad infinitum*, and that hope was as extravagant as fear. How was he to foretell that the French people, like the man in the fable, would kill, in their frantic eagerness, the fine goose he had brought to lay them so many golden eggs? His fate was like that which may be supposed to have overtaken the first adventurous boatman who rowed from Erie to Ontario. Broad and smooth was the river on which he embarked; rapid and pleasant was his progress; and who was to stay him in his career? Alas for him! the cataract was nigh. He saw, when it was too late, that the tide which wafted him so joyously along was a tide of destruction; and when he endeavoured to retrace his way, he found that the current was too strong for his weak efforts to stem, and that he drew nearer every instant to the tremendous falls. Down he went over the sharp rocks, and the waters with him. *He* was dashed to pieces with his bark, but the waters, maddened and turned to foam by the rough descent, only boiled and bubbled for a time, and then flowed on again as smoothly as ever. Just so it was with Law and the French people. He was the boatman, and they were the waters.

In 1716, the finances of the country of France were in a state of the utmost disorder. A profuse and corrupt monarch, whose profuseness and corruption were imitated by almost every functionary, from the highest to the lowest grade, had brought France to the verge of ruin. The national debt amounted to 3000 millions of livres, the revenue to 145 millions, and the expenses of government to 142 millions per annum; leaving only three millions to pay the interest upon 3000 millions.

In the midst of this financial confusion Law appeared upon the scene. No man felt more deeply than the regent the deplorable state of the country, but no man could be more averse from putting his shoulders manfully to the wheel. He disliked business; he signed official documents without proper examination, and trusted to others what he should have undertaken himself. The cares inseparable from his high office were burdensome to him. He saw that something was necessary to be done; but he lacked the energy to do it, and had not virtue enough to sacrifice his ease and his pleasures in the attempt. No wonder that, with this character, he listened favourably to the mighty projects, so easy of execution, of the clever adventurer whom he had formerly known, and whose talents he appreciated.

When Law presented himself at court he was most cordially received. He offered two memorials to the regent, in which he set forth the evils that had befallen France, owing to an insufficient currency, at different times depreciated. He asserted that a metallic currency, unaided by a paper money, was wholly inadequate to the wants of a commercial country, and particularly cited the examples of Great Britain and Holland to shew the advantages of paper. He used many sound arguments on the subject of credit, and proposed as a means of restoring that of Prance, then at so low an ebb among the nations, that he should be allowed to set up a bank, which should have the management of the royal revenues, and issue notes both on that and on landed security. He further proposed that this bank should be administered in the king's name, but subject to the control of commissioners to be named by the States-General.

While these memorials were under consideration, Law translated into French his essay on money and trade, and used every means to extend through the nation his renown as a financier. He soon became talked of. The confidants of the regent spread abroad his praise, and every one expected great things of Monsieur Lass. On the 5th of May, 1716, a royal edict was published, by which Law was authorised, in conjunction with his brother, to establish a bank under the name of Law and Company.

4. It can be inferred that the author views Law:
- **A** as a buffoonish figure who intended no harm but caused catastrophe through his foolishness.
- **B** as a daring and unique man who ultimately used his knowledge of economics for unscrupulous ends.
- **C** as a credulous man who was taken in by the people he associated with.
- **D** as an unwittingly tragic figure who caused catastrophe without meaning to.

5. It can be concluded that the financial disaster can be blamed on all of the following except:
- **A** the regent's unwillingness to take on the duties of his position.
- **B** the French citizens' and officials' unawareness of how markets and currency worked.
- **C** the French officials' unwillingness to question Law's ideas
- **D** the French desperation for a solution to their fiscal problems.

6. Based on the passage, we can infer that the rest of this chapter will:
- **A** provide a detailed pro and con discussion of whether Law was fully responsible for the crash.
- **B** explain the principles of banking and investment that were at play in Law's story.
- **C** give a detailed account of how various people's actions brought Law's bank down.
- **D** critique Law's bank as an institution that was untenable according to modern knowledge of finance.

7. It can be inferred from the passage that the scheme failed because:
- **A** the system of paper money did not work and led to runaway inflation.
- **B** people lacked confidence in Law's ideas and hoarded coins rather than switching to paper money, leading to a crash.
- **C** people invested in Law's scheme in the hope of making fortunes, then sold en masse when their assets turned out to be valueless.
- **D** people turned against Law due to his reputation as a scoundrel and refused to invest or put money in his bank.

Questions 8 – 10

The following compilation of crime percentages were based on some Thailand research in relation to other countries of the Western world.

Table 1. Crimes Statistics: Thailand and selected Western Countries

Assaults (per thousand people)	Burglaries (per thousand people)
US 7.6	Australia 21.7
UK 7.5	UK 13.8
Canada 7.1	Canada 8.9
Australia 7.0	US 7.1
France 1.8	France 6.1
Germany 1.4	Japan 2.3
Thailand 0.3	Thailand 0.2
Japan 0.3	Germany N/A

Rapes (per hundred thousand people)	Gun Murders (per hundred thousand people)
Australia 79	Thailand 31
Canada 73	US 2.8
US 30	Canada 0.5
UK 14	Germany 0.5
France 14	Australia 0.1
Germany 9	UK 0.1
Thailand 6	Japan N/A
Japan 2	France N/A

8. The number of violent crimes (listed as Assaults, Rapes, and Murders) were committed in Australia and Thailand in this selected temporal frame. Which country had the LEAST amount of violent crimes listed?
   A Japan
   B Thailand
   C France
   D Germany

9. Which country would define the closest approximation to a mean or average of the crime of rape listed?
   A Germany
   B US
   C UK
   D France

10. The main purpose of the chart provided could be inferred to:
   A assess Thailand's crime rates in relation to other countries.
   B promote gun control measures or legislation in Thailand.
   C provide statistics for analysis in Thailand's violent and non-violent crimes.
   D compare and contrast the different crimes worldwide in relation to Thailand.

UNIT 4

Questions 11 – 13

The 20th century saw a thriving automobile industry. By the mid 1900s, mass production of cars significantly contributed to a dependence of international trade on the petroleum industry.

The following cartoons pertain to the present impact of petrol (gasoline) on politics and economy.

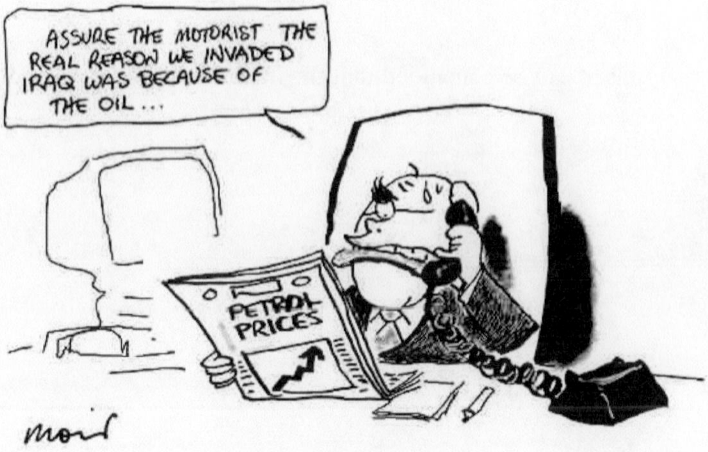

Cartoon I

11. The cartoon conveys that oil:
- **A** dictates global events.
- **B** is used as an excuse for war.
- **C** is highly important for motorists.
- **D** affects political and economic affairs.

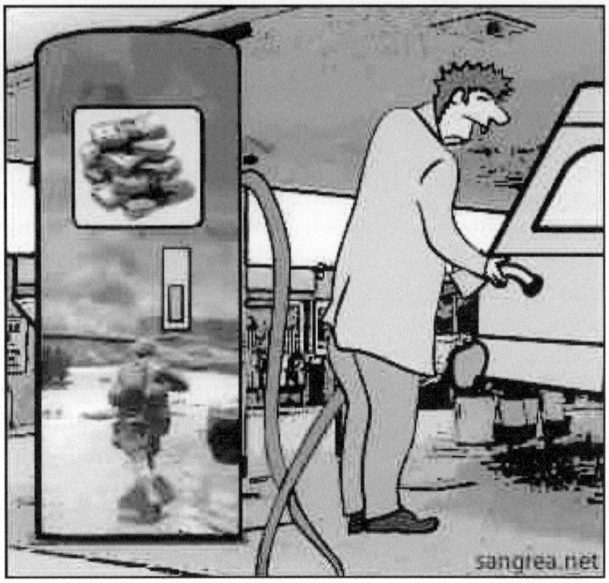

Cartoon II

12. Cartoon II portrays, in a relatively unfavourable light:

I. the petrol gas station
II. the car owner.
III. the petrol company.
IV. the government.

A I and II
B I, II, III, and IV
C I and III
D I, II, and III

13. Based on the two cartoons, it can be concluded that the impact of oil in world politics and economy is:
A disastrous.
B unpleasant.
C self-defeating.
D megalomaniac.

UNIT 5

Questions 14 – 16

The following passage discusses how language affects the interpretation of results in a social research.

In a recent article written by Mary Sykes, she discusses the mystification of class issues as written about by a British organisation, the Community Relations Commission (CRC) that is concerned about racial and economic disparities. The focus of Sykes' article is to point out how the ambiguity in the CRC's language distorts the causes of poverty, homelessness, and other social problems facing the lower class. Sykes argue that the result of this language is that minorities (economically or racially disadvantaged people) are easily perceived as both passive recipients of nameless forces rather than as active members of a racist, classist society, and as ultimately to blame for their predicament.

At one point in her article, Sykes identifies how many people are referred to in the CRC's report, how many times they are listed, and what sorts of verbs they are associated with. In this case there are only three: 'parents', 'young minorities', and 'the Commons Select Committee'. Parents and the CSC are referred to once; young minorities are referred to 14 times. Young minorities are connected to very few active verbs. They are said to 'drift from place to place' and to 'drift into petty crime'. In other words, they are perceived as passive participants who do not control their interaction with their environment.

Sykes also examines what social and institutional processes might cause the homelessness of young blacks. She finds that there is nothing specific mentioned, only vague entities such as 'a complex world', 'social problems', and 'problems of individual and ethnic identity'. She then turns to individual people that may act as catalysts or links in the causal chain. The article states that young minorities get in trouble 'at home, at work, and at school', but no mention is made of parents, bosses, teachers, or police. The reader is left to fill in the steps that lead from 'problems of ethnic identity' to homelessness, since there are no variables -neither institutions nor humans -- to link together, or even to suggest how to link together, vague entities like 'social problems' and the specific group of young minorities.

It is clear why Sykes worries that a reader may blame the victims. Specifying other forces that contribute to problems would dilute the concentration of references to young minorities, and make it clear that the causal chain leading to such predicaments as homelessness is made up of many links. This is important because while some readers may adequately fill in the gaps, others will not have the presupposed knowledge necessary to make connections to other people and institutions. More important, they will not be able to question these factors, since they do not even know what they are. From Sykes' analysis of the passage it appears that, on the one hand, victims are blameless; they are completely passive and inert participants. On the other hand, there are no other specified causal factors at work, so the black youths become the only participants.

Sykes' article demonstrates the power that language has over our perceptions of others. However, her argument might be more powerful had she conducted a study to note the difference in people's perception of young minorities based on the CRC passage and one that plentifully cited specific causes. This neglect can detract from her conclusion, because although she shows effectively a possible reading of the CRC report, she does not follow this up by showing that the article actually does affect people in her hypothesised way.

14. Sykes provides examples such as 'a complex world', 'social problems', and 'problems of individual and ethnic identity' to explain that:

A the CRC does not use enough verbs when describing links in the causal chain.
B CRC is too ambiguous in stating what actual events affect the outcome.
C CRC is intentionally distorting information.
D CRC is unaware of what the actual causes are.

15. Which of the following statements best sums up the contradiction Sykes claims lies in the CRC's report?

A Young minorities are responsible for both their situation and responsible for the more general 'social problems'.
B Young minorities are both passive victims and responsible participants.
C Young minorities are the victims of social institutions yet these social institutions take on no specific form.
D Young minorities are both passive, and they are victims of social and institutional processes.

16. The article written by Mary Sykes does NOT resemble a study:

A showing that smoking causes cancer, citing evidence of a high incidence of smokers having lung cancer.
B showing that smoking causes cancer, citing evidence that relatively few cases of lung cancer are found in non-smokers.
C arguing that violence on TV increases actual violence, citing evidence that a strong correlation exists between watching TV and committing violent acts.
D arguing that violence on TV increases actual violence, citing evidence that people who view violent TV programs commit more violent acts than those who do not view violent TV programs.

UNIT 6

Questions 17 – 22

The following passage is adapted from an article written by Mikhal Dekel in 2014 for the Nineteenth-century Gender Studies Journal.

The central romance in *Pride and Prejudice* begins when Mr. Darcy refuses to dance in an unfamiliar social setting. His explanation of his behaviour—"I detest it unless I am particularly acquainted with my partner"—has been interpreted by generations of readers as the excuse of a man with "ten thousand a year" who reeks of class privilege and indifference to social inferiors. Some hundred pages later, Mr. Darcy repeats his confession saying, "I am ill qualified to recommend myself to strangers." Hearing this, Elizabeth Bennet addresses her reply to Darcy's cousin Colonel Fitzwilliam. "Shall we ask him," she queries, "why a man of sense and education, and who has lived in the world, is ill qualified to recommend himself to strangers?" Fitzwilliam tells her, "It is because he will not give himself the trouble."

Darcy's own reason is quite different. "I certainly have not the talent which some people possess of conversing easily with those I have never seen before. I cannot catch their tone of conversation, or appear interested in their concerns, as I often see done." Here too, readers, like the characters with whom Darcy is conversing, perceive his reply as an expression of class privilege. This essay asks what happens to our understanding of Darcy and Elizabeth if we take Darcy at his word, i.e., we accept that he really cannot easily decipher social interactions. It asks, more specifically, what happens to our understanding of these characters if we read Darcy's social inadequacy as a product of disability rather than an individual choice. How does such a reading affect our perceptions of Darcy, Elizabeth and the novel in general if we interpret Darcy's self-presentation literally rather than ironically? Further, what becomes of the larger issues traditionally understood as the novel's main concerns: relations between genders and classes, women's growth and autonomy, the pitfalls and triumphs of communication? And what happens if we interpret a novelistic character through the lens of neurology over (or in addition to) the lens of class and gender difference?

To begin with, such a reading would mark a radical shift in the critical tradition of *Pride and Prejudice*, which has been grounded for nearly two centuries in the assumption that Darcy's behaviour is a product of agency and choice; this is how Darcy is also regarded within the novel's world: by Elizabeth Bennet, by Colonel Fitzwilliam and by nearly every other character in the novel. But what if we were to make the opposite assumption: that Darcy's social awkwardness is owed to an organic condition which is at least in part outside his control? This relatively narrow question raises many larger ones, some of which have begun to be addressed by Lisa Zunshine, Ellen Spolsky, Alan Richardson, Blakey Vermeule and other humanistic scholars working on biosocial approaches to literature.

Nineteenth century novels, Austen's in particular, have provided excellent raw material for the discussion of these approaches. Austen's protracted, leisurely explorations of characters' affective and cognitive states within their cultural environments seemingly reveal, as Kay Young writes, a "modern, post-Cartesian conception of the integrated mind – as cognitive, affective, embodied and relational." This engagement with the nature of mind and consciousness in Austen's novels is not incidental to her plots; rather, as Palmer and Richardson have shown, Austen's slowly evolving plots allow for a serious interrogation of the nature of mind and brain, including its various "types" and constitutions.

Taking the works of these critics as my starting point, I will present in what follows a triple-tiered argument. First, I will argue that the quality of Darcy's social communication can and should be read through the lens of disability; more specifically, I will argue that Darcy's characterisation is that of a man on the mild side of the autistic spectrum. Secondly, I will use this understanding of Darcy's character, particularly in relation to the character of Elizabeth Bennet, to interrogate the idea of the spectrum and consider the impact this possibility may have on contemporary literary theory. Thirdly, I will treat the gendered aspect of what has come to be termed "neurodiversity" and look at the ways in which taking autism into account may reshape feminist theory and how feminist theory, in turn, can help us think of autism in more compassionate and productive ways. In particular I will argue that the recent turn to emotions in humanistic and social study, coupled with current research on the pliability of the brain and its inter-related nature, can help us form more generous ideas about both gender differences and social-emotional disability.

17. This passage contrasts which two possible approaches to literature?
- **A** Gender criticism versus apolitical close reading
- **B** Psychological reading versus readings based on structure and form
- **C** Freudian readings versus readings based on modern ideas about psychology
- **D** Gender and class-based readings versus cognitive readings

18. In lines 1 - 6, the passage assumes that most readers do which of the following when reading literature?
- **A** Analyse character statements to learn the reasons behind their actions
- **B** Analyse character behaviour for clues to the characters' innate cognitive strengths and weaknesses.
- **C** Analyse character behaviour as clues to the character's goodness and moral worth
- **D** Analyse author statements about characters for clues about their true nature

19. The author's argument would be most strongly thrown into question by an article arguing that:
- **A** the character of Darcy in *Pride and Prejudice* is one of many in literature who lacks conventional social skills and show autistic-like behaviour.
- **B** the character of Darcy in *Pride and Prejudice* has privileges from his gender and inherited wealth that greatly outweigh any disadvantages he suffers from a psychological condition.
- **C** analysing literature in terms of neurology is compatible with analysing it in terms of gender, race and class, since all these factors affect a person's behaviour.
- **D** autism can only be determined by a diagnosis from a medical health professional because many people self-report autistic-like symptoms.

20. Lines 41 - 45 use the term 'post-Cartesian'. Based on surrounding context, what does it mean to see the mind in a 'Cartesian' way?
- **A** To see it as an organic organ subject to disease and decay
- **B** To see it as a faculty separate from the physical body within which it exists
- **C** To see it as a social construct based on a given culture's expectations of what a mind should do
- **D** To see it as having little capacity for understanding others' mental states in social situations

21. Which of the following would not count as a "biosocial approach" to criticism?

- **A** A critic discussing a detective novel in which all the suspects are lying, and examining the strains this puts on the detective's ability to infer their mental states
- **B** An art critic analysing how pointillist paintings make use of the brain's mechanisms for perceiving colour
- **C** A critic examining how the arbitrary fact of a character's skin colour affects her experiences and the way other characters treat her
- **D** An analysis of how self-referential fictions take advantage of the brain's natural tendency to become absorbed in a fiction in order to create humour

22. Which of the following pieces of evidence from elsewhere in the article most strongly supports the claim that "Darcy's characterisation is that of a man on the mild side of the autistic spectrum" (lines 53 - 54)?

- **A** "From Darcy's very first appearance in the novel, at the Netherfield ball, his social behaviour is described as giving offence to others ('he was the proudest, most disagreeable man in the world, and every body hoped that he would never come there again')."
- **B** "Other characters may be caricatured as snobs who intend to humiliate, but Darcy's speech seems to simply lack in elasticity, emotional subtlety and social awareness."
- **C** "Even before Elizabeth answers, the narrator concludes that Darcy's delivery [of a marriage proposal] 'was unlikely to recommend his suit.'"
- **D** "The term Autism is first mentioned in a 1943 paper titled 'Autistic Disturbances of the Affective Contact," by the pediatric neurologist Leon Kanner. In this paper, Kanner discusses case studies of eleven children [who] present impairment in social and communicative skills."

UNIT 7

Questions 23 – 24

"You can lead a horse to water, but you can't make it drink."

English proverb

23. This statement equates the notion that:

- **A** trying to do two things at once will make you fail in both.
- **B** what seems easy is impossible to achieve.
- **C** just as distance tests a horse's strength, time reveals a person's character.
- **D** people, like horses, will only do what they will.

"Seek wisdom like a beggar."

Burmese Proverb

24. This proverb implies that:

- **A** wisdom is often deceiving.
- **B** a wise person speaks less.
- **C** attaining wisdom requires humility.
- **D** a wise person is indifferent to material wealth.

Question 25

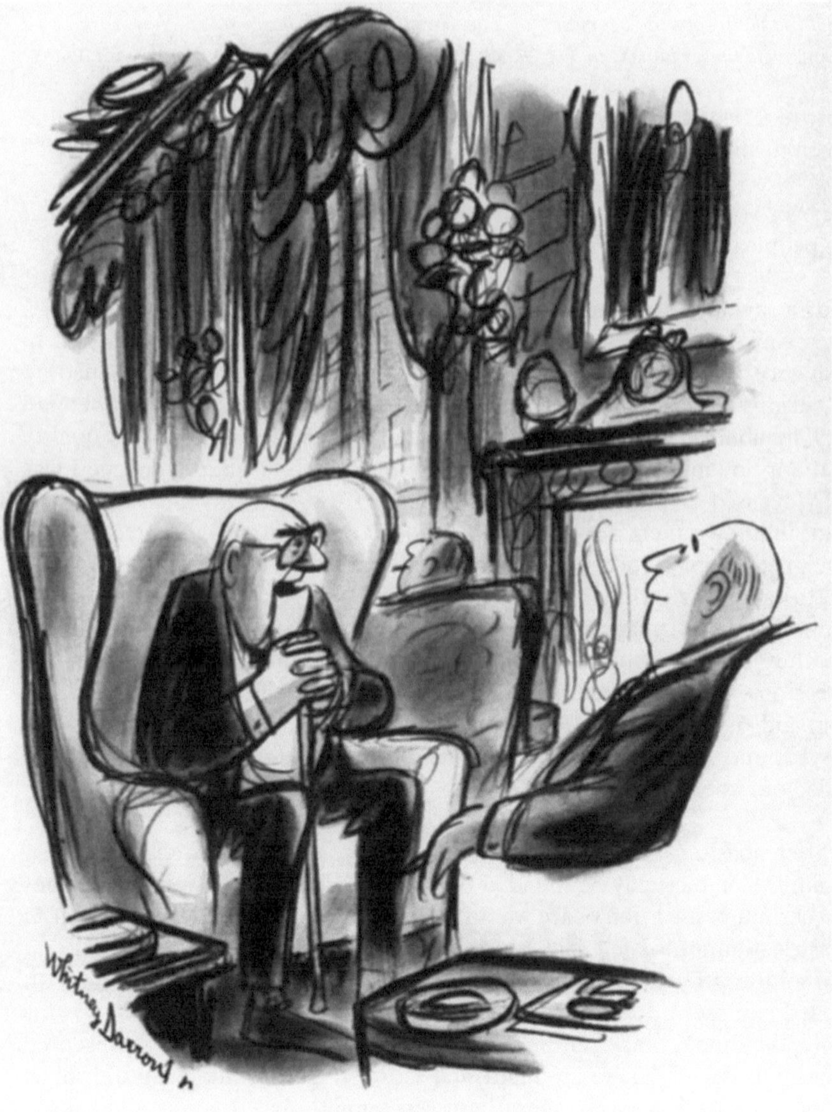

"I'm rich, yes, but not rich beyond my wildest dreams."

Used with permission. Credit: Whitney Darrow, Jr./The New Yorker Collection/The Cartoon Bank.

25. Which of the following would best describe the theme of this cartoon?

A He who is not contented with what he has, would not be contented with what he would like to have.

B Greed is a bottomless pit which exhausts the person in an endless effort to satisfy the need without ever reaching satisfaction.

C Greed is a fat demon with a small mouth and whatever you feed it is never enough.

D Wealth is like sea-water; the more we drink, the thirstier we become.

Questions 26 – 30

The following extract is taken from the beginning of ***The Great Gatsby****, a novel set in New York in 1922. It is narrated by Nick Carraway, a young man who moves in next to Jay Gatsby and subsequently becomes friends with him.*

In my younger and more vulnerable years my father gave me some advice that I've been turning over in my mind ever since.

"Whenever you feel like criticising any one," he told me, "just remember that all the people in this world haven't had the advantages that you've had."

He didn't say any more but we've always been unusually communicative in a reserved way, and I understood that he meant a great deal more than that. In consequence I'm inclined to reserve all judgments, a habit that has opened up many curious natures to me and also made me the victim of not a few veteran bores. The abnormal mind is quick to detect and attach itself to this quality when it appears in a normal person, and so it came about that in college I was unjustly accused of being a politician, because I was privy to the secret griefs of wild, unknown men. Most of the confidences were unsought--frequently I have feigned sleep, preoccupation, or a hostile levity when I realised by some unmistakable sign that an intimate revelation was quivering on the horizon--for the intimate revelations of young men or at least the terms in which they express them are usually plagiaristic and marred by obvious suppressions. Reserving judgments is a matter of infinite hope. I am still a little afraid of missing something if I forget that, as my father snobbishly suggested, and I snobbishly repeat, a sense of the fundamental decencies is parcelled out unequally at birth.

And, after boasting this way of my tolerance, I come to the admission that it has a limit. Conduct may be founded on the hard rock or the wet marshes but after a certain point I don't care what it's founded on. When I came back from the East last autumn I felt that I wanted the world to be in uniform and at a sort of moral attention forever; I wanted no more riotous excursions with privileged glimpses into the human heart. Only Gatsby, the man who gives his name to this book, was exempt from my reaction--Gatsby who represented everything for which I have an unaffected scorn. If personality is an unbroken series of successful gestures, then there was something gorgeous about him, some heightened sensitivity to the promises of life, as if he were related to one of those intricate machines that register earthquakes ten thousand miles away. This responsiveness had nothing to do with that flabby impressionability which is dignified under the name of the "creative temperament"--it was an extraordinary gift for hope, a romantic readiness such as I have never found in any other person and which it is not likely I shall ever find again. No--Gatsby turned out all right at the end; it is what preyed on Gatsby, what foul dust floated in the wake of his dreams that temporarily closed out my interest in the abortive sorrows and short-winded elations of men.

26. Which of the following phrases does not align with the phrase: 'whenever you feel like criticising any one, just remember that all the people in this world haven't had the advantages that you've had' (lines 3-4)?

A Be kind, for everyone is fighting a battle you know nothing about.
B It is always ridiculous to imagine yourself superior to other people.
C What separates privilege from entitlement is gratitude.
D Privilege is invisible to those who have it.

27. In lines 19 - 20, Nick says he sometimes forgets that 'fundamental decencies are parcelled out unequally at birth'. What does this reveal about his character?

A He often overlooks his own privilege.
B He expects everyone to have the same opportunities as he does.
C He doesn't understand why others aren't as 'decent' as him.
D He is privileged to the point of ignorance.

28. From the way he is presented by the narrator, what word might be used to describe Gatsby?

A Virtuous
B Auspicious
C Faultless
D Ostentatious

29. From this extract, what can we glean about the relationship between Nick and Gatsby?

A Nick is attracted to Gatsby.
B Nick wants to model himself after Gatsby.
C Nick is jealous of Gatsby.
D Nick is in awe of Gatsby.

30. What is the tone of the extract?

A Pensive
B Reflective
C Nostalgic
D Analytical

Questions 31 – 36

Preludes

I

The winter evening settles down
With smell of steaks in passageways.
Six o'clock.
The burnt-out ends of smoky days.
And now a gusty shower wraps
The grimy scraps
Of withered leaves about your feet
And newspapers from vacant lots;
The showers beat
On broken blinds and chimney-pots,
And at the corner of the street
A lonely cab-horse steams and stamps.
And then the lighting of the lamps.

II

The morning comes to consciousness
Of faint stale smells of beer
From the sawdust-trampled street
With all its muddy feet that press
To early coffee-stands.

With the other masquerades
That time resumes,
One thinks of all the hands
That are raising dingy shades
In a thousand furnished rooms.

III

You tossed a blanket from the bed,
You lay upon your back, and waited;
You dozed, and watched the night revealing
The thousand sordid images
Of which your soul was constituted;
They flickered against the ceiling.
And when all the world came back
And the light crept up between the shutters,
And you heard the sparrows in the gutters,
You had such a vision of the street
As the street hardly understands;
Sitting along the bed's edge, where
You curled the papers from your hair,
Or clasped the yellow soles of feet
In the palms of both soiled hands.

IV

His soul stretched tight across the skies
That fade behind a city block,
Or trampled by insistent feet

At four and five and six o'clock
And short square fingers stuffing pipes,
And evening newspapers, and eyes
Assured of certain certainties,
The conscience of a blackened street
Impatient to assume the world.

I am moved by fancies that are curled
Around these images, and cling:
The notion of some infinitely gentle
Infinitely suffering thing.

Wipe your hand across your mouth, and laugh;
The worlds revolve like ancient women
Gathering fuel in vacant lots.

-T.S. Eliot

31. Why is the title "Preludes" significant?
A Each section serves to introduce the next.
B Each section has a beginning, followed by an ending.
C Each section refers to something about to happen.
D Each section introduces a main idea.

32. In the penultimate, "the notion of some infinitely gentle / Infinitely suffering thing" (lines 50 – 51) refers to:
A human compassion
B fanciful interests.
C human soul.
D human frailty.

33. The tone of the poem is:
A melancholic.
B brooding.
C nonchalant.
D disinterested.

34. In relation to the theme, the images of the poem are made up of:
A daily rituals.
B insignificant details.
C motivating clues.
D secular trivialities.

35. Two ideas are juxtaposed. Which of the following ratios would be the best answer?
A Sacred and profane
B Spiritual and mundane
C Ritualised and indifferent
D Secular and misanthropic

36. "The conscience of a blackened street / Impatient to assume the world" (lines 46 – 47) means:
A really no conscience, a masquerade.
B burdened with trivial matters, in a hurry.
C a conscience based on hastiness.
D an emotionally bereft concern with time.

Questions 37 – 40

The following two poems are reminiscences of the respective writers' medical-related experiences.

I. The Look on Your Face

Your skin pale with worry,
your mouth a straight line,
the fear in your eyes--
all this told me,
more than the nausea,
more than the fact that I couldn't move my head,
that something was really wrong.

You thought I wouldn't see.

I looked up at the ceiling,
at its pattern of dots,
white, and brighter white,
that could mean anything, or nothing,
but that kept me from thinking
about the look on your face,
before you had time to rearrange it
into a mask of hope.

Priscilla Mainardi

II. What's Left Over

One and a half tubes of smörgåskaviar[1], most
of a jar of blueberry jam, a full jar of lingonberries.
Four sets of blue plaid pajamas--God forbid
I should have gotten him red. Six pairs
of reading glasses, going back
in five-year increments. Hearing-aid
batteries stashed by the lamp.
Three packages of adult diapers.
Our marriage certificate.
The rest of the morphine.

Ruth Bavetta

[1]Smörgåskaviar: a fish roe spread eaten in Scandinavia and Finland

37. Which of the following emotions best describe each poem?

	Poem I	Poem II
A	hope	resignation
B	denial	acceptance
C	confusion	loss
D	courage	passivity

38. In reading Poem I, the word 'hope' in the last line emphasises the speaker's feeling of:

A discomfort.
B contempt.
C distrust.
D anxiety.

39. Lines 4 - 8 in Poem II suggests which of the following states of health?

A Recovery
B Remission
C Deterioration
D Death

40. Line 11 in Poem I and lines 3 - 4 in Poem II commonly refer to colours as a means to:

A relive memories.
B distract emotions.
C conceal anxiety.
D alleviate pain.

Questions 41 – 46

The following excerpt was adapted from a research article published in the International and Multidisciplinary Journal of Social Sciences in July 2015.

Prior to the industrial revolution the pursuit of leisure activities was the prerogative of the elite and wealthy. The contemporary concept of leisure as "time spent not working" is a product of social and economic changes in the 19th century associated with the industrial revolution in Europe and North America. The combination of political emancipation and the expansion of the franchise, the reduction of both the working day and the length of the working week, along with rising standards of living, enabled greater numbers of people to engage in other activities, including leisure activities.

The way leisure is defined is highly 'context-dependent', especially in Western industrialised societies where leisure is influenced by the wider economy, the way work is organised, the political system and the decline of community in the 20th century. There was a further expansion of this leisure time, accompanied by rising standards of living, in the second half of the 20th century.

What people did with leisure time was influenced by technological changes in the media and the entertainment sectors. During the 19th century the mechanisation of print expanded the production of newspapers, books and magazines. A rise in literacy levels meant reading in the home increased.

In the 20th century there was an evolution in new forms of media—cinema, radio and television—and a merging of some aspects of those media. The expansion of cinema at the turn of the century was part of the transition to increasingly visual forms of communication. In the 1920s radio became more widespread, and in the next decade sound and image merged in films. The introduction of radio increased the amount of entertainment available in the home in the 1920s, a trend that intensified with the rapid uptake of television in the 1960s. During the 1990s the migration of the computer from work to personal use also had an impact on leisure. A decade later mobile phones and tablets made media more available for personal use.

In contemporary emerging societies a rapid social transition, similar to that which occurred in Western industrialised societies in the 19th and 20th centuries, took place starting in the 1970s. Today, with the globalisation of the media and technology, it is possible for these groups to leapfrog stages of technological development and engage with the latest media technologies available. These technological changes are completely revolutionising how people spend their leisure time in all societies.

Because leisure has social and economic implications, it became an important area of research in the 20th century, and of interest to governments. Leisure is an important economic activity. In Britain leisure accounted for between 25% and 38% of consumer spending and is an important form of employment. The OECD report measuring leisure has identified three key criteria for defining leisure: time, activities and states of mind. The economic determinants of leisure focus on 'residual time not spent in paid work'.

Leisure is also defined in terms of the allocation of time in the adult life cycle, and time-use studies are used to document activities when people are in work and away from work. Trends in all OECD countries from 1970-2005 indicated that, contrary to general perceptions, time spent working was not increasing except for certain groups. The greatest reduction in work hours in recent decades occurred in the 1970s. Average hours in paid work in OECD countries were 1595 hours a year, though averages differed considerably between countries. The reduction in work hours has not translated into an increase in leisure hours. The OECD study used four criteria for defining time: 1. leisure (using the 'narrow' definition—low levels' of personal care—45% of time) 2. paid work 3. unpaid work 4. personal care (including sleep) and 5. 'other'. Gender, age, social class, race/ethnicity and employment status are all important influences on the time available for leisure and how people engage with technology in their leisure. Older age groups have more leisure time once taking care of young children ceases, and in almost all countries men have more leisure time than women, whether using a 'broad' definition (factors in a high level of personal care) or the narrow definition. Employed married women with dependent children have the least time for leisure. Those with lower incomes may have to work longer hours or have more than one job, which may decrease leisure time.

41. The passage implies which of the following about leisure and personal care?

- **A** Leisure and personal care should be considered the same thing since both involve time not spent working.
- **B** Some activities can be defined variously as leisure or as personal care.
- **C** Personal care is a form of work because it is essential to performing job-based activities, whereas leisure is optional.
- **D** Both leisure and personal care were concepts that did not exist in earlier time periods.

42. Which hypothetical piece of evidence would most strongly undermine the author's argument in the passage?

- **A** A study showing that when people have more free time, their amount of leisure stays the same because they spend more time on childcare and housework
- **B** A study showing that leisure is becoming less satisfying as people spend more time browsing the internet and less time socialising
- **C** A study showing that activities that were once considered leisure activities are now classed in other categories by most people
- **D** A study showing that working people in past centuries spent just as much time relaxing and socialising outside of work as today's people, although they lacked the concept of 'leisure activities'

43. Based on passage information, which invention would we expect to have altered the way people use their leisure time?

- **A** The answering machine
- **B** The shopping mall
- **C** The VCR
- **D** The interstate highway system

44. According to passage information, which of the following is not a potential reason that the 'reduction in work hours has not translated into an increase in leisure hours'?

- **A** Parents now spend more time on childcare than they did in previous decades.
- **B** When people's time at work decreases, they spend more time sleeping and grooming.
- **C** The population overall has gotten younger.
- **D** For every increase in leisure, more workers are needed in the entertainment and hospitality industries.

45. Based on passage information, we can expect which of the following to happen in future decades?

- **A** People will have fewer children in order to reap the benefit of more free time.
- **B** People worldwide will spend more leisure time engaged with personal electronic devices rather than socialising with the wider community.
- **C** Leisure time will continue to increase in western countries as time spent working continues to decrease.
- **D** The definition of leisure time will change.

46. Imagine a person is cooking a meal for their family. According to passage information, this could be categorised differently depending on if:

- **A** the meal is more elaborate and time-consuming to prepare than necessary.
- **B** the person regards cooking as a hobby rather than a task necessary for survival.
- **C** the person has sufficient free time outside of work to cook the meal and engage in other enjoyable activities outside of work hours.
- **D** the person is socialising with a friend while cooking the meal.

Question 47

The rise of new technologies has led to more choices in how people want to consume information. We can pick between paper books, e-books, read on our computer, phone, or tablet screens, or choose to consume our favorite book in an audio version without having to engage in reading at all.

This has led to a stream of research that investigates how those various ways of consuming information influence our attention and how we process information. A study was conducted at the University of Waterloo to find out how the mind responds to reading material presented in different ways. Participants had to read three different passages. One was read silently, because this is perceived as the most common way of processing written information. In addition to that the participants had to listen to an audio recording and read a passage aloud. For each encounter, mind wandering was probed by asking the participants if they had been mind-wandering or not. After each passage, participants were asked to rate their interest on a five-point scale, and their memory was tested with a multiple-choice comprehension test. The results are displayed in the following table.

	Sample 1		Sample 2	
Encounter type	**Memory**	**Interest**	**Memory**	**Interest**
READING ALOUD				
Mind wandering	−0.08	−0.20*	0.01	−0.36***
Memory		0.14		0.23*
READING SILENTLY				
Mind wandering	−0.36***	−0.43***	−0.22*	−0.42***
Memory		0.40***		0.33***
LISTENING				
Mind wandering	−0.25**	−0.51***	−0.43***	−0.65***
Memory		0.33***		0.43***

****$p < 0.001$, ***$p = 0.01$, *$p < 0.05$.*

Table 1 Pearson Product-Moment Correlations of Proportion of Mind Wandering (Mind Wandering), Memory Test Proportion Correct (Memory), and Interest Rating (Interest), for Each Encounter Type and Sample

Source: Adapted from T.L. Varao Sousa, J.S.A. Carriere, and D. Smilek, "The Way We Encounter Reading Material Influences How Frequently We Mind Wander." Copyright 2013 Perception Science.

47. Which hypothesis is best supported by the data from Table 1?

A Reading aloud is the best way of preventing mind wandering.
B Reading aloud is the best way of enhancing memory performance.
C Listening is the best way of enhancing memory performance.
D Listening is the best way of preventing mind wandering.

UNIT 14

Questions 48 – 54

The Englishman and Music

Englishmen have never cared for music as they care for football or film stars. They like singing, most of them, either making a noise themselves or listening to others. There is a long tradition both of religion and conviviality by which men and women who would not claim to be musical will gladly take part in a hymn or join in a chorus. There has been a tradition centuries old by which choral singing in parts has been a fairly widespread pastime. In Elizabethan times, it was something more: for about forty years it appears to have been a fashionable craze among cultivated people, and, though it is easy to overestimate the excellence of their performance, the singers of those days conferred an incalculable benefit upon the art of music and a rich heritage upon English musical life by their assiduous practice, thereby stimulating to activity a whole school of first-rate composers. Assuredly England has never been a "land without music", as the reproachful German phrase went a couple of generations ago. But music, musical affairs, musical politics, new compositions, the status of individual artists, have never in this country been "front page news": the bulk of the population does not really care how music gets along provided that on occasion it can obtain what it wants for ceremonial occasions, for occasional polite entertainment, for lubricating the wheels on which its theatrical or restaurant entertainment runs . . . Our festivals, our opera seasons, and the performance of our virtuosi, even our musical competitions, leave our national phlegm unmoved. The tantrums of a prima donna have a certain human interest for our popular newspapers, but by and large the great public does not care. Are we then a musical people?

. . . Are we a blue-eyed people? Some of us are blue-eyed and some of us are musical. The musical enthusiasts are a small minority, but the potentially musical are a much larger number. Perhaps five percent are definitely insusceptible to music . . . The rest are capable of having their interest, and perhaps ultimately their love, aroused for the art. There are many things in this beautiful world that compete for our attention, for our limited time, for our not unlimited mental energy, and for our pocket-money, and many will sacrifice music to fly-fishing or watching birds . . . many a gifted person with artistic abilities that run in several directions at once will devote himself to water-colours instead of the piano. But the coming of the wireless broadcasting has at least made numbers of people, running into the hundreds of thousands, aware of music as a factor in their experience of life.

The kind of satisfaction that comes from music . . . is one of the things that give value to life. Possibly it is the most perfect example of those higher disinterested values that give significance to life, in that it is unmixed with social, political and ethical purposes and so provides us with an instance of what is valuable in and for itself alone without further object. Not everyone will want this particular kind of satisfaction from music; some take a more hedonistic view of it and value it as just one more ingredient in the good life. Still others are content with the opiate of light music. But whichever of the many sorts of psychological satisfaction that can be getting from music may be found by any individual, it is so far a part of his life's experience, and more and more people are coming to be aware of it as such and to value it as an enrichment of their lives.

Adapted from Frank Howes, Fontana Guide to Orchestral Music, 8 1958 by Collins Clear Type Press

48. According to the passage, the attitude of the English during the Elizabethan era was most influential in resulting to:

A an interest in musical affairs which had never been there previously.
B increased participation in hymn and choir singing in churches.
C a revival in choral singing in parts.
D great musical compositions by a new era of composers.

49. The author rhetorically asks "Are we a blue-eyed people?" in order to:

A exemplify that nearly half of the population is, at least, partially musical.
B convey the irrelevance of questioning whether the English are musical or not.
C affirm that, as a whole, the English are a musical people.
D emphasise the contrasting attitudes towards music between the English, Germans and Russians.

50. The passage suggests that the English might be less interested than the Germans in news concerning:

A football and the newest developments in that sport.
B issues in musical entertainment that might affect business.
C outdoor hobbies.
D developments in the music and theatre industry.

51. According to the author, someone who is "insusceptible to music" is someone who:

A is uninterested in musical affairs, musical politics, and the state of individual artists.
B would rather not waste their time fly-fishing or bird-watching.
C is incapable of having their interest for music aroused.
D would rather devote their time to water-colours.

52. The passage indicates that the renewed musical awareness in England can in part be attributed to:

A the assiduous practicing of singers over the years.
B the introduction of wireless broadcasting into society.
C the emergence of a whole new school for talented composers.
D a decline of interest in football that has occurred over the years.

53. Based on the passage, one could conclude that the author believes that music's greatest value lies in the fact that:

A it has a great ability to bring joy.
B it is a form of expression which is detached from politics, social and cultural issues.
C it is a component of the good life.
D it has the power to enrich the life of every individual who becomes aware of it.

54. Which of the following would be the best reason why the English are NOT musically inclined as other Germanic countries?

A They are more interested in hobbies and sports.
B They have no great composers, in relation to Bach or Beethoven.
C Look at modern culture, such as the British invasion of Rock and Roll.
D Their musical proclivities are in the nascent stages of development.

UNIT 15

Questions 55 – 58

The following are two short passages from Shakespeare (Macbeth and King Lear).

Macbeth, after his queen's death, makes the following famous speech in Act 5, Scene 5, lines 17-28.

MACBETH: Wherefore was that cry?

SEYTON: The queen, my lord, is dead.

MACBETH: She should have died hereafter;
There would have been a time for such a word.
To-morrow, and to-morrow, and to-morrow,
Creeps in this petty pace from day to day
To the last syllable of recorded time,
And all our yesterdays have lighted fools

The way to dusty death. Out, out, brief candle!
Life's but a walking shadow, a poor player
That struts and frets his hour upon the stage
And then is heard no more: it is a tale
Told by an idiot, full of sound and fury,
Signifying nothing

Act III, Scene IV, during the terrible storm. While his fool takes shelter in a hovel, Lear, after learning of his daughter's treachery, throws himself into the wilderness, losing his sanity or so it seems. Here he remains standing for a moment in the rain and meditates on the poor citizens of his kingdom:

Poor naked wretches, whereso'er you are,
That bide the pelting of this pitiless storm,
How shall your houseless heads and unfed sides,
Your loop'd and window'd raggedness, defend you
From seasons such as these? O, I have ta'en
Too little care of this! Take physic, pomp;
Expose thyself to feel what wretches feel,
That thou mayst shake the superflux to them,
And show the heavens more just.

55. In the Macbeth passage, the tonality of Shakespeare suggests:
A remorse.
B despair.
C grief.
D anxiety

56. In the King Lear passage, the tonality of Shakespeare suggests:
A shattered innocence.
B profound enlightenment.
C remorseful compassion.
D indignant defiance.

57. In the passage from King Lear "Take Physic, pomp" is a strange and anachronistic utterance. Based on the context of the passage, this would mean in modern day language:
A to understand the poor's suffering.
B to feel the elements of the storm arrogantly.
C to strive to make things just.
D pompous men take a taste of this medicine.

58. Which of the following generalisations could be inferred concerning both passages?
A Life is unjust.
B Life is meaningless.
C Life is constantly changing.
D Life is storm-like.

Questions 59 – 62

The following are pictures from World War 1 and World War 2.

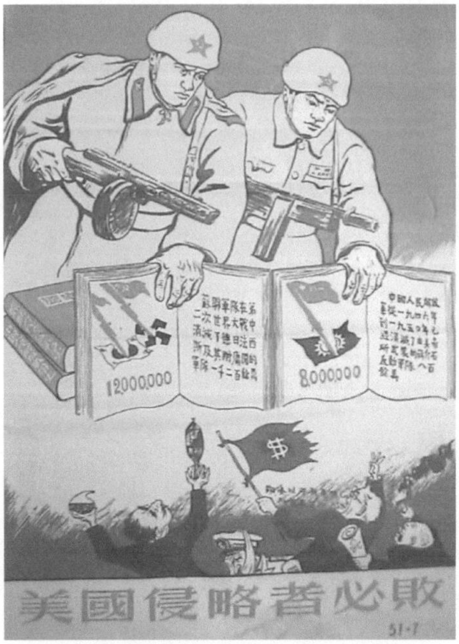

Picture 1–from China ("You will be defeated!" - translation)

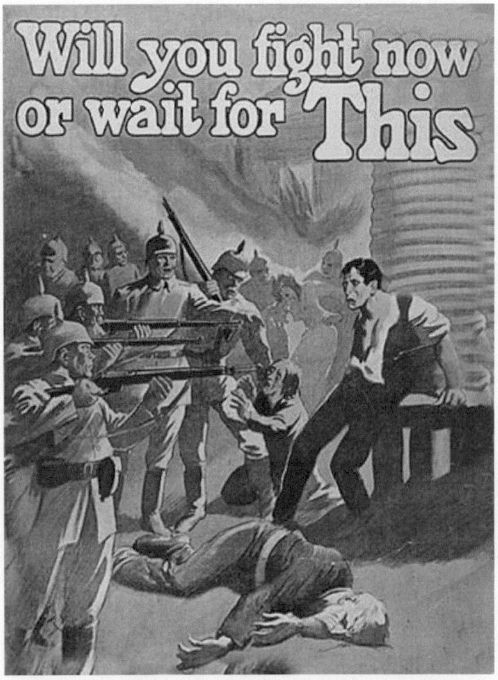

Picture 2–from Australia (WW1)

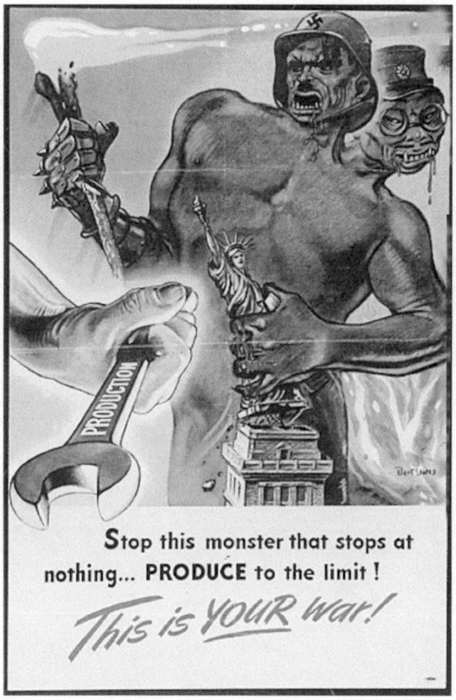

Picture 3–from the U.S.

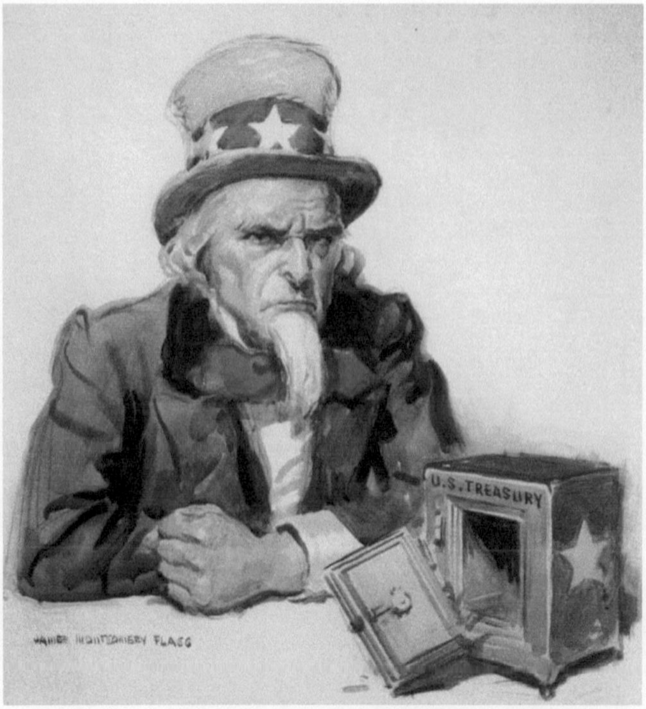

Picture 4–from the U.S.

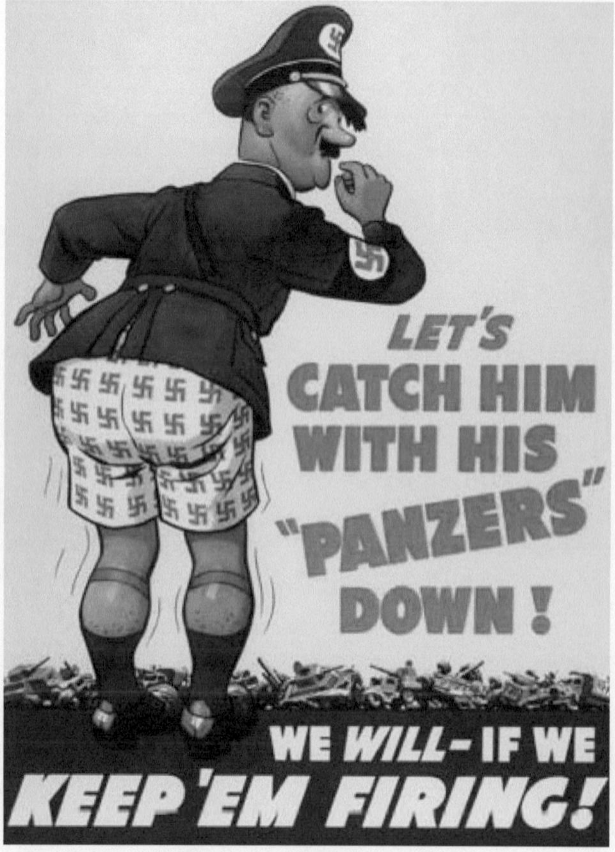

Picture 5–from the UK

It can be argued that all of the 5 pictures represent propaganda to at least some extent.

59. Which of the pictures appeals mostly to a "sense of patriotism and homeland"?
- **A** 1
- **B** 5
- **C** 3
- **D** 2

60. Which of the following ratios depict the representations' use of emotional appeals respectively (1-5)?
- **A** Quantity, quality, labour, taxes, derision
- **B** Rage, sentiment, workers, money, laughter
- **C** Intimidation, fear, demonisation, economic insecurity, humour
- **D** Polarisation, patriotism, caricatures, foolhardiness

61. Which picture is the most emotionally charged?
- **A** 3
- **B** 4
- **C** 1
- **D** 5

62. Which picture "polarises"? (either/or thinking)
- **A** 2
- **B** 5
- **C** 1
- **D** 3

CANDIDATE'S NAME ______________________________ BOOKLET GS1-III

STUDENT ID ______________________________

GAMSAT Masters Series Test 3

Reasoning in Humanities and Social Sciences

Questions: 1-62
Time: 100 minutes

INSTRUCTIONS: Of the 62 questions in this test, many are organised into groups preceded by stimulus material. After evaluating the stimulus material, select the best answer to each question in the group. Some questions are independent of any descriptive passage or each other. Similarly, select the best answer to these questions. If you are unsure of an answer, eliminate the alternatives that you know to be incorrect and select an answer from the remaining alternatives. To indicate your selection, use a pencil to circle the letter in your test booklet. If you wish to make notes, you may use two A4 sheets as scratch paper since this will be provided to you on test day for the new, digital GAMSAT (some test centres permit the use of whiteboards). No marks are deducted for wrong answers.

The Gold Standard GAMSAT* has been designed exclusively to test knowledge and thinking skills. The exam may contain hypothetical statements and/or express controversial ideas. Statements contained herein do not necessarily reflect the policy, position, or view of RuveneCo Inc.

OPEN BOOKLET ONLY WHEN TIMER IS READY.

Answers and worked solutions are available to the original owner at gamsat-prep.com.
(register at: www.gamsat-prep.com/gamsat-humanities-and-social-sciences)

UNIT 1

Questions 1 – 10

On August 23, 1998, UNESCO commemorated the first International Day for the Remembrance of the Slave Trade and its Abolition. By December 9 of the following year, the City Council of Liverpool passed a motion that acknowledged and apologised for its responsibility in participating in a three century-old trade that significantly marked in the history of Africa. Ten years later, the United States Senate issued an apologetic statement dated June 18, 2009 criticising the "fundamental injustice, cruelty, brutality, and inhumanity of slavery".

The following passages are related views on the African Slave Trade and its abolition in 1807.

View I

Slavery had long existed in Africa even before the British landed the continent. Tribal wars turned captured prisoners into either domestic servants or Black slaves bought by Arabs and neighbouring traders in the Near East.

Africans did not see the arrival of the Europeans as trouble. Many native rulers and British traders maintained a symbiotic relationship that lasted for more than 300 years. African suppliers compensated for the Europeans' lack of familiarity of the continent's interiors, providing tens of millions of people shipped to the New World. In exchange, Europeans exposed the African elite to the culture of a fast-changing civilisation. Children of African royalties voyaged to Europe to acquire Western sophistication. Back home, many African kings and slavers acquired fortune and power enjoying refined and technologically advanced articles like hats, bracelets, textiles, sheepskin gloves, swords, knives, alcohol, guns and gunpowder.

Concurrently, the steady supply of African labourers in the different sugar colonies of Britain contributed to the growth of the burgeoning commercial trade in sugar and rum. When the slave trade was formalised in 1672, Britain can be said to have engaged in a moral venture because they were saving captured Africans - who may otherwise have been ordered to be executed in tribal courts – and, at the same time, boosting the European trade.

1. View I argues that:
- **A** African rulers were as much responsible as the Europeans for advancing the slave trade.
- **B** Africa had a crude slavery system before the Europeans came.
- **C** the slave trade brought cultural and economic benefits to Africa's society.
- **D** slave trade did not significantly alter the situation of the African slaves.

2. Based on View I, the nature of the British-African slave trade was characterised by:
- **A** diplomacy.
- **B** cultural exchange.
- **C** humanitarianism.
- **D** expediency.

View II

Debates have recently arisen pertaining to demands in the Unites States for reparations for those centuries of unpaid African slave labour: At the height of the triangular slave trade between Britain, Africa and America during the 17th century, two-thirds of African slaves were sold by either native or European slavers to the Americas to work in sugar and cotton plantations. They became "properties" of plantation owners in a system called chattel slavery. This meant that they were not paid as labourers and that their statuses as slaves became inherited bondages passed on to their offspring. Men toiled in the fields or mines; women worked outdoors or in the master's home; children, depending on their capacity at the time, did domestic chores like fetching water or weeding. The European slave owners and traders made tremendous profits out of free African labour during the height of the sugar, coffee and tobacco commerce in Europe.

In an article published online by Abayomi Azikiwe, editor of Pan-African News Wire, the following opinion was expressed regarding the admission of certain large American corporations in their involvement in the exploitative slave system: "Yet this admission is inadequate without efforts to correct the historical damage done to the people who have still not reclaimed their rightful place within modern society. Only with the overthrow of capitalism and imperialism and the seizure of the wealth stolen by the capitalists can true reparations be granted to the African people."

3. The opinion stated in View II suggests that the demand for reparations emphasises:

A how the slave trade brought adversities to the African race.
B how the most profitable institutions gained their wealth through the slave trade.
C how the slave trade robbed African people of their worth in society.
D the significant contribution of the slave trade to world trade.

4. According to the passage, being a slave meant becoming a part of the owner's:

A family estate.
B inventory.
C labour force.
D household charge.

View III

The slave trade reshaped, if not reversed, the meaning that members of African societies gave to the word "slavery" and more significantly, the way they perceived their place in the world. The natives lived in constant fear of being seized and herded away to oblivion, never to return. The lingering threat in safety and survival felt by the natives, as well as the captured slaves, further propelled them to seek salvation from spirits and gods. Some Africans who managed to seek refuge in the deep interiors believed that white people took slaves to eat them. Slaves and their descendants, if ever they survived the harsh conditions in plantation camps, lived to regard themselves as inferior members of society.

5. According to View III, "slavery" for the African natives became equated with:

A death.
B inferiority.
C social phobia.
D superstition.

View IV

Historian-philosopher Thomas Kuhn views the social sciences to be characterised by a "tradition of claims, counterclaims, and debates over fundamentals." Changes in the assessment of and sensitivities to key social issues are oft-times influenced by the very events surrounding them throughout history.

The general perception of slavery, for instance, was once dictated by cultural factors: ideas propagated by the "White benevolence" gave the Renaissance merchant limitless permission to enslave African "savages" in the name of civilisation. Public response, however, shifted when late 18th century abolitionists campaigned for "equality of races" and "freedom for all" in the light of democracy. The abolition of the slave trade thus transformed the general understanding of slavery from cultural to political.

Modern historians now identify the Transatlantic Trade as an exploitative enterprise that used an existing local custom of trading human captives to gain economic advantage in the free trade. Radical writers even regard the modern worker to be slaves themselves. "The only difference is that slaves are now paid and are given a wider leverage of personal freedom in the disguised term of workers."

6. The term "workers" was used as a point of comparison in View IV to emphasise that:

A slavery has never been abolished.
B slavery is motivated by pecuniary advantage.
C workers are treated better than slaves.
D workers benefit from the business chain while slaves do not.

7. What connotation do the terms "cultural' and "political" have in common?
   - **A** The idea of slavery changes, consistent to its historical milieu.
   - **B** The idea of slavery was always dealt with altruistic justifications.
   - **C** Despite changes in the perception of slavery, economic interests remain as the driving force behind its practice.
   - **D** Slavery has always been a complex historical issue.

Questions 8 – 10 refer to Views I to IV.

8. Based on the opinions expressed in Views I to IV, had not the Europeans endeavoured in the slave trade:
   - **A** the African natives would have engaged in the business with other merchants for as long as there was a continued demand for slaves.
   - **B** the African natives would have remained secluded from world civilisation.
   - **C** Africa would have achieved national development.
   - **D** Africans would have enjoyed equal rights and opportunities as free people in Europe and America.

9. Which among the 4 views would favour an admission of guilt and granting of reparations by Europe and America?
   - **A** I and II
   - **B** II and III
   - **C** II and IV
   - **D** IV only

10. Views I to IV recognise the fact that:
   - **A** Africans were as morally depraved as the Europeans who bought slaves from them.
   - **B** since the arrival of the Europeans, Africans have been denied many rights.
   - **C** the motive behind the slave trade is commercialism.
   - **D** slavery is an undeniable component of human society.

UNIT 2

Questions 11 – 12

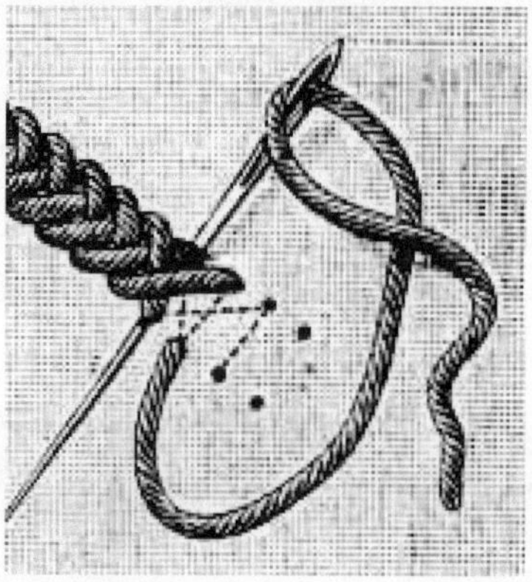

The Basket Stitch is one of the numerous stitching styles in sewing. It is a solid border stitch, which is worked between two lines, giving a raised effect with the use of a stout thread. Below is a modified diagram on how to work this decorative pattern.

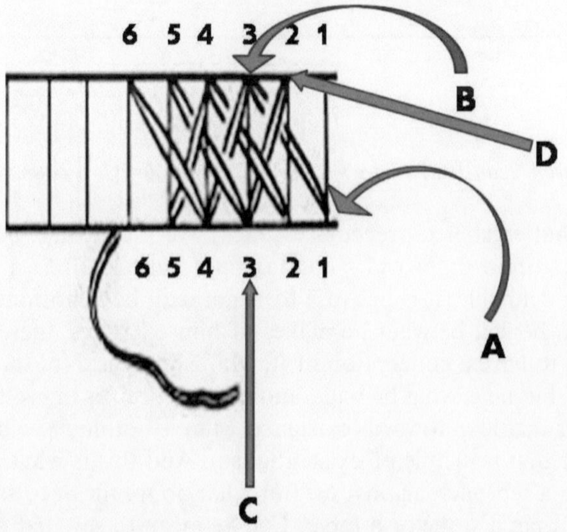

Mark two parallel lines and dot at even distances on both lines.

A. Insert the needle from under to the upper side of the cloth on the first dot of the lower line.
B. Cross over and insert in the third dot on the top line.
C. Bring it out on the opposite dot on the lower line.
D. Put the needle into the second dot on the top line, bring out on the second dot on the lower line, and cross over to dot four.

Continue the pattern until the end of the worked area on the cloth.

11. An alternate use of this stitching style is mostly likely NOT associated with:
A basket weaving.
B cross-stitching.
C patchwork.
D mending.

12. Based on the diagram, Dot 5 on the upper line likely follows:
A pattern B: cross-over, under insertion.
B pattern B: cross-over, upper insertion.
C pattern D: cross-over, under insertion.
D pattern D: cross-over, upper insertion.

UNIT 3

Questions 13 – 17

The following passage is an excerpt from Jean-Paul Sartre's lecture, Existentialism is a Humanism.

What do we mean by saying that existence precedes essence? We mean that man first of all exists, encounters himself, surges up in the world — and defines himself afterwards. If man as the existentialist sees him is not definable, it is because to begin with he is nothing. He will not be anything until later, and then he will be what he makes of himself. Thus, there is no human nature, because there is no God to have a conception of it. Man simply is. Not that he is simply what he conceives himself to be, but he is what he wills, and as he conceives himself after already existing — as he wills to be after that leap towards existence. Man is nothing else but that which he makes of himself. That is the first principle of existentialism. And this is what people call its "subjectivity," using the word as a reproach against us. But what do we mean to say by this, but that man is of a greater dignity than a stone or a table? For we mean to say that man primarily exists — that man is, before all else, something which propels itself towards a future and is aware that it is doing so. Man is, indeed, a project which possesses a subjective life, instead of being a kind of moss, or a fungus or a cauliflower. Before that projection of the self nothing exists; not even in the heaven of intelligence: man will only attain existence when he is what he purposes to be. Not, however, what he may wish to be. For what we usually understand by wishing or willing is a conscious decision taken — much more often than not — after we have made ourselves what we are. I may wish to join a party, to write a book or to marry — but in such a case what is usually called my will is probably a manifestation of a prior and more spontaneous decision. If, however, it is true that existence is prior to essence, man is responsible for what he is. Thus, the first effect of existentialism is that it puts every man in possession of himself as he is, and places the entire responsibility for his existence squarely upon his own shoulders. And, when we say that man is responsible for himself, we do not mean that he is responsible only for his own individuality, but that he is responsible for all men. The word "subjectivism" is to be understood in two senses, and our adversaries play upon only one of them. Subjectivism means, on the one hand, the freedom of the individual subject and, on the other, that man cannot pass beyond human subjectivity. It is the latter which is the deeper meaning of existentialism. When we say that man chooses himself, we do mean that every one of us must choose himself; but by that we also mean that in choosing for himself he chooses for all men. For in effect, of all the actions a man may take in order to create himself as he wills to be, there is not one which is not creative, at the same time, of an image of man such as he believes he ought to be. To choose between this or that is at the same time to affirm the value of that which is chosen; for we are unable ever to choose the worse. What we choose is always the better; and nothing can be better for us unless it is better for all. If, moreover, existence precedes essence and we will to exist at the same time as we fashion our image, that image is valid for all and for the entire epoch in which we find ourselves. Our responsibility is thus much greater than we had supposed, for it concerns mankind as a whole.

13. In this passage, the author's discussion is intended to:

A explicate the principles of his philosophical movement.
B inveigle sceptical views towards his philosophy.
C counter accusations posed against his philosophical views.
D compare and contrast existence and essence.

14. Existence is introduced in the passage as a(n):

A destiny.
B volition.
C prerequisite.
D experience.

15. According to Sartre, "subjectivity" (lines 25 – 28) constitutes:

A recognising the value of one's choice and how this would affect the world.
B the ability to choose one's destiny and change mankind
C a coextensive responsibility over one's individual freedom and over humanity.
D a spontaneous decision to realise one's place in the world.

16. The author suggests that being human means having the capacity to:

A choose the quality of one's life.
B make a positive contribution to the world.
C realise one's destiny.
D make responsible choices.

17. In line 5, "there is no human nature, because there is no God to have a conception of it" means that:

A man will exist, whether or not God exists.
B even if God existed, man will continue to make choices.
C no external force can save man from his irresponsible choices.
D only man creates his own destiny.

UNIT 4

Questions 18 – 24

This unit contains two views of the woman's role in society.

PASSAGE I

At the present time, when women are beginning to take part in the affairs of the world, it is still a world that belongs to men – they have no doubt of it at all and women have scarcely any. To decline to be the Other, to refuse to be a party to the deal – this would be for women to renounce all the advantages conferred upon them by their alliance with the superior caste. Man-the-sovereign will provide woman-the-liege with material protection and will undertake the moral justification of her existence; thus she can evade at once both economic risk and the metaphysical risk of a liberty in which ends and aims must be contrived without assistance. Indeed, along with the ethical urge of each individual to affirm his subjective existence, there is also the temptation to forgo liberty and become a thing. This is an inauspicious road, for he who takes it – passive, lost, ruined – becomes henceforth the creature of another's will, frustrated in his transcendence and deprived of every value. But it is an easy road; on it one avoids the strain involved in undertaking an authentic existence. When man makes of woman the Other, he may, then, expect to manifest deep-seated tendencies towards complicity. Thus, woman may fail to lay claim to the status of subject because she lacks definite resources, because she feels the necessary bond that ties her to man regardless of reciprocity, and because she is often very well pleased with her role as the Other.

- From Woman as Other, Simone de Beauvoir

18. For de Beauvoir, the relationship that transpires between man and woman is that of:

A a master to his slave.
B provider and dependant respectively.
C conspiracy.
D communal partnership.

19. The author suggests that the roles of men and women are dictated by:

A survival needs.
B social preconditions.
C male orientation.
D personal motives.

20. According to de Beauvoir, the woman considers herself as:

A a willing subordinate of man.
B an outsider in man's world.
C an insecure social being.
D man's moral responsibility.

PASSAGE II

At the present stage of history civilisation is almost exclusively masculine, a civilisation of power, in which woman has been thrust aside in the shade. Therefore it has lost its balance and it is moving by hopping from war to war. Its motive forces are the forces of destruction, and its ceremonials are carried through by an appalling number of human sacrifices. This one-sided civilisation is crashing along a series of catastrophes at a tremendous speed because of its one-sidedness. And at last the time has arrived when woman must step in and impart her life rhythm to this reckless movement of power.

For woman's function is the passive function of the soil, which not only helps the tree to grow but keeps its growth within limits. The tree must have life's adventure and send up and spread out its branches on all sides, but all its deeper bonds of relation are hidden and held firm in the soil and this helps it to live. Our civilisation must also have its passive elements broad and deep and stable. It must not be mere growth but harmony of growth. It must not be all tune but it must have its time also. This time is not a barrier, it is what the banks are to the river; they guide into permanence the current which otherwise would lose itself in the amorphousness of morass. It is rhythm, the rhythm which does not check the world's movements but leads them into truth and beauty.

- From Woman, Rabindranath Tagore

21. Tagore views the relationship of man and woman as:

A one-sided.
B narcissistic.
C a pair of opposing forces.
D destroyer and pacifier, respectively.

22. The passage suggests that the author considers the woman as:

A dormant.
B the better sex.
C the stabilising mate of man.
D the embodiment of truth and beauty.

23. Compared to Tagore's, male power according to de Beauvoir is:

A constructive.
B manipulative.
C dependent on the woman.
D superior to the woman.

24. The views of Tagore and de Beauvoir are primarily similar in:

A indicating that man's power is dependent on the woman's passivity.
B recognising that the woman's role is defined by the male point of view.
C perceiving the crucial function of the woman in society.
D the way they view the subtle power of the woman.

UNIT 5

Questions 25 – 28

The following passage forms part of the climax of the play A Woman of No Importance by Oscar Wilde. Mrs. Arbuthnot, the female character to whom the title "A Woman of No Importance" pertains, has admitted to her son, Gerald, that he is a child born out of wedlock.

MRS. ARBUTHNOT. Men don't understand what mothers are. I am no different from other women except in the wrong done me and the wrong I did, and my very heavy punishments and great disgrace. And yet, to bear you I had to look on death. To nurture you I had to wrestle with it. Death fought with me for you. All women have to fight with death to keep their children. Death, being childless, wants our children from us. Gerald, when you were naked I clothed you, when you were hungry I gave you food. Night and day all that long winter I tended you. No office is too mean, no care too lowly for the thing we women love - and oh! how I loved you. Not Hannah, Samuel more. And you needed love, for you were weakly, and only love could have kept you alive. Only love can keep any one alive. And boys are careless often and without thinking give pain, and we always fancy that when they come to man's estate and know us better they will repay us. But it is not so. The world draws them from our side, and they make friends with whom they are happier than they are with us, and have amusements from which we are barred, and interests that are not ours: and they are unjust to us often, for when they find life bitter they blame us for it, and when they find it sweet we do not taste its sweetness with them. . . You made many friends and went into their houses and were glad with them, and I, knowing my secret, did not dare to follow, but stayed at home and closed the door, shut out the sun and sat in darkness. What should I have done in honest households? My past was ever with me. . . And you thought I didn't care for the pleasant things of life. I tell you I longed for them, but did not dare to touch them, feeling I had no right. You thought I was happier working amongst the poor. That was my mission, you imagined. It was not, but where else was I to go? The sick do not ask if the hand that smooths their pillow is pure, nor the dying care if the lips that touch their brow have known the kiss of sin. It was you I thought of all the time; I gave to them the love you did not need: lavished on them a love that was not theirs. . . And you thought I spent too much of my time in going to Church, and in Church duties. But where else could I turn? God's house is the only house where sinners are made welcome, and you were always in my heart, Gerald, too much in my heart. For, though day after day, at morn or evensong, I have knelt in God's house, I have never repented of my sin. How could I repent of my sin when you, my love, were its fruit! Even now that you are bitter to me I cannot repent. I do not. You are more to me than innocence. I would rather be your mother - Oh! Much rather! - than have been always pure. . . Oh, don't you see? Don't you understand? It is my dishonour that has made you so dear to me. It is my disgrace that has bound you so closely to me. It is the price I paid for you - the price of soul and body - that makes me love you as I do. Oh, don't ask me to do this horrible thing. Child of my shame, be still the child of my shame!

25. Mrs. Arbuthnot's remark, "Men don't understand what mothers are" (line 1), implies that she expects men:

A do not care about a mother's concerns.
B are emotionally detached from their mothers.
C have different views on love and pleasure than women.
D are naturally drawn into worldly pursuits.

26. Mrs. Arbuthnot opted to devote her services to the Church because she:

A wanted to conceal her past.
B had nowhere to go.
C was seeking absolution for her past sins.
D felt accepted and useful in this circle.

27. The tone of this excerpt is:

- **A** repentant.
- **B** bitter.
- **C** regretful.
- **D** imploring.

28. Which of the following approximates the meaning of lines 31-32, "It is the price I paid for you – the price of soul and body – that makes me love you as I do"?

- **A** You know it's love when you want to give joy and damn the consequences.
- **B** Love is always an investment.
- **C** It is love alone that gives worth to all things.
- **D** Even shameful love carries a pride.

UNIT 6

Questions 29 – 30

The following cartoon relates to the 2004 National Mental Health Report in Australia acknowledging the fact that there is a lack of mental health services in the public system. As a result, only patients who pose an immediate threat to themselves or others are committed.

In reaction, a number of doctors had to overstate the patients' symptoms and secure a mental health order in order to get them into the community centres.

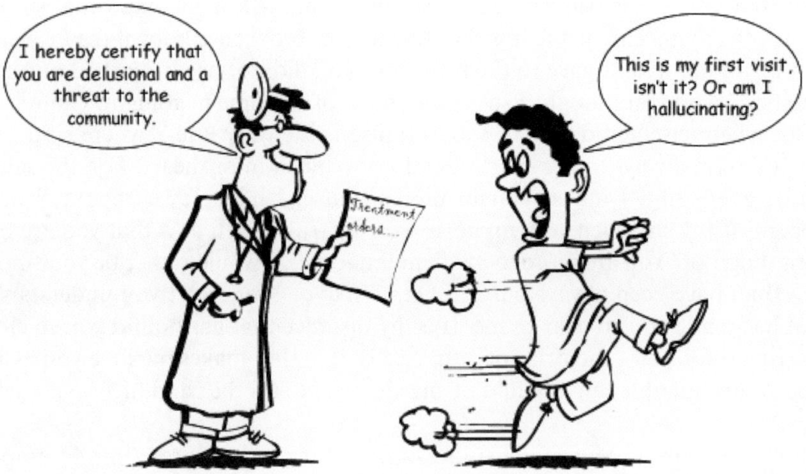

29. Based on the cartoon, the patient's reaction indicates that he:

- **A** is truly suffering from hallucinations.
- **B** doubts the doctor's diagnosis.
- **C** is confused about his own mental state.
- **D** has finally confirmed his true mental condition in lieu of the doctor's statement.

30. The cartoon implies that exaggerating the patient's symptoms:

- **A** confuses the patient.
- **B** deceives the patient.
- **C** justifies the moral obligation of medical doctors.
- **D** compromises the doctor's liability to his patient.

Questions 31 – 36

The following is a writer's analysis of various theories of personality.

Personality theorists view life in terms of varying models. One of these, the "conflict model," portrays humans as inextricably caught in the opposition of two great forces, producing a psychological conflict that is experienced as an uncomfortable state of tension and anxiety. The exact nature of these opposing forces varies with different theorists. Jung, for example, conceived of both forces as residing within the self—one is derived from the worldly, practical goals of the conscious mind, and the other emerges from the ancient communal memories of the collective unconscious. Freud, on the other hand, attributed only one of the forces to the individual. This was the complex of selfish, pleasure-seeking drives, which he called the "id." The opposing force, for Freud, originated in the altruistic and cooperative goals of society; although he believed that this force became internalised during childhood into the part of the personality he named the "superego." Whatever the version of the conflict model, personal adjustment is defined as a successful compromise between the urgings of these two unalterable forces and an ensuing reduction in tension. Maladjustment is thought to occur when the individual leans too heavily toward one or the other of the forces and ignores the claims of the opposing force.

A second basic personality model, called the "fulfilment model," posits the existence of only one, rather than two great life forces. Neither conflict nor compromise is considered inevitable under this model, and the subjective experience of tension is given a positive interpretation. Life is viewed as the unfolding of the great life force, with the experience of pleasurable tension (e.g. enthusiasm, excitement) being heightened by a vigorous expression of this force. In the version of the fulfilment model evolved by Maslow, the life force is conceptualised as the realisation of one's own unique inherent capabilities, or self-actualisation. Other fulfilment theorists, such as Fromm, see the life force as promoting the expression of universal human capabilities or striving toward cultural ideals. In no version of the fulfilment model is there a conflict between the true interests of the individual and the social group: both are best served by vigorous striving that transcends the conventional. Such lifestyles, however, may come into conflict with the immediate social context, which often contains inhuman and punitive elements. Individual maladjustment is thought to arise when a person suppresses the life force in order to live in complete conformity with his or her social context.

Yet a third personality model is also well represented among modern personality theorists. This is the "consistency model." It is qualitatively different from either of the preceding models in that it does not stress the specific content of personality or inherent forces. Rather, it focuses on the importance of congruence, or fit, between thinking and reality. Consistency theory presents humans as scientists who are constantly observing and mapping the world. The pieces of the map—our ideas about the world—are termed "cognitions" by Kelley and "expectations" by McClelland. It is hypothesised that gaps between these ideas about the world and the evidence of our sensory perceptions generate tension and anxiety, motivating humans to strive for a congruent set of cognitions that match observations of the real world as nearly as possible. Maladjustment is seen in terms of poor maps that distort or deny aspects of the real world.

While it is difficult to conduct experiments that test the validity of most aspects of these models, the tension reduction component of the theories can be investigated. Behaviourists, who generally conceptualise learning as occurring in response to tension reduction, have carried out a considerable amount of relevant experimentation. According to behaviourists, learning is the establishment of a bond between a particular stimulus and a particular response, this learned link becomes established when the response brings about a decrease in the level of tension existing in the organism. (The decrease in tension is called a reward or reinforcement.) However, while the behaviourist tension-reduction model appears to apply in many learning situations, learning can apparently also take place without such a tension-reducing reward. Experimentally, this has been shown to occur in "latent learning," where learning takes place without reward and appears in the form of changed behaviour at some later time.

Other experimental evidence refuting the hypothesis that behaviour is always" motivated by tension reduction includes findings that primates attempting to solve "intellectual" problems sometimes work to the point of developing ulcers. Also, research on sensory deprivation has shown that when humans are deprived of their usual sensory stimulation, they strongly seek such stimulation.

31. According to the passage, Freud's and Jung's theories of human personality:

A disagree on the basic causes of maladjustment in human beings.
B disagree on the role of tension-reduction as a motivator of human behaviour.
C agree on the definition of the id and superego, but disagree on their roles.
D agree that tension derives from a failure to attain a successful compromise between conflicting forces.

32. The "fulfilment model" implies that:

A maladjustment results from a denial of basic cultural ideals.
B the inevitability of compromise and conflict are denied.
C mental conflict is a necessary consequence of a vigorous expression of the life force.
D all the fulfilment theorists agree on the nature of the one great force.

33. The following statements are true about the consistency model:

I. Maladjustment is seen as a conceptual distortion of the real world.
II. Cognitions or expectations are thought to play a central role in human behaviour.
III. Perceptions contribute to the formulation and revision of cognitions or expectations.
IV. The definitions of cognitions and expectations are similar to Freud's definition of the id construct.

A II and IV
B I, II, III
C II only
D II, III and IV

34. Based on the passage, maladjustment could be generally viewed as conflicting psychological forces that:

A cause tension and anxiety within the individual.
B affect the way an individual behaves or responds to systems in society.
C upsets the way an individual interprets reality.
D suppresses the freedom of an individual to express his or her real nature.

35. Which of the following personality theories would closely represent a compromise of tension forces in the individual in the statement "I believe in the magic of love"?

A Jung's theory on worldly goals of the conscious mind versus the collective unconscious
B Freud's theory on the selfish, pleasure-seeking "id" versus the altruistic "superego"
C Maslow's theory on self-actualisation
D Fromm's theory on the expression of the universal ideals

36. In correlating the tension-reduction model of the behaviourists, what would be the best reward to an individual with the consistency model's personality?

A Social Acceptance
B Affirmation
C Tolerance
D Recognition

UNIT 8

Questions 37 – 42

The following passage discusses the differences between the theatrical stage and the silent film (referred in the excerpt as photoplay) from The Art of the Moving Picture by Vachel Lindsay.

When the veteran stage-producer as a beginning photoplay producer tries to give us a dialogue in the motion pictures, he makes it so dull no one follows. He does not realise that his camera-born opportunity to magnify persons and things instantly, to interweave them as actors on one level, to alternate scenes at the slightest whim, are the big substitutes for dialogue. By alternating scenes rapidly, flash after flash: cottage, field, mountain-top, field, mountain-top, cottage, we have a conversation between three places rather than three persons. By alternating the picture of a man and the check he is forging, we have his soliloquy. When two people talk to each other, it is by lifting and lowering objects rather than their voices. The collector presents a bill: the adventurer shows him the door. The boy plucks a rose: the girl accepts it. Moving objects, not moving lips, make the words of the photoplay.

. . . It was a theatrical sin when the old-fashioned stage actor was rendered unimportant by his scenery. But the motion picture actor is but the mood of the mob or the landscape or the department store behind him, reduced to a single hieroglyphic.

The stage-interior is large. The motion-picture interior is small. The stage out-of-door scene is at best artificial and little and is generally at rest, or its movement is tainted with artificiality. The waves dash, but not dashingly, the water flows, but not flowingly. The motion picture out-of-door scene is as big as the universe. And only pictures of the Sahara are without magnificent motion.

The photoplay is as far from the stage on the one hand as it is from the novel on the other. Its nearest analogy in literature is, perhaps, the short story, or the lyric poem. The key-words of the stage are passion and character; of the photoplay, splendour and speed. The stage in its greatest power deals with pity for some one especially unfortunate, with whom we grow well acquainted; with some private revenge against some particular despoiler; traces the beginning and culmination of joy based on the gratification of some preference, or love for some person, whose charm is all his own. The drama is concerned with the slow, inevitable approaches to these intensities. On the other hand, the motion picture, though often appearing to deal with these things, as a matter of fact uses substitutes, many of which have been listed. But to review: its first substitute is the excitement of speed-mania stretched on the framework of an obvious plot. Or it deals with delicate informal anecdote as the short story does, or fairy legerdemain, or patriotic banners, or great surging mobs of the proletariat, or big scenic outlooks, or miraculous beings made visible.

And the further it gets from Euripides, Ibsen, Shakespeare, or Molière—the more it becomes like a mural painting from which flashes of lightning come—the more it realises its genius. Men like Gordon Craig and Granville Barker are almost wasting their genius on the theatre. The Splendour Photoplays are the great outlet for their type of imagination.

The typical stage performance is from two hours and a half upward. The movie show generally lasts five reels, that is, an hour and forty minutes. And it should last but three reels, that is, an hour. Edgar Poe said there was no such thing as a long poem. There is certainly no such thing as a long moving picture masterpiece.

The stage-production depends most largely upon the power of the actors, the movie show upon the genius of the producer. The performers and the dumb objects are on equal terms in his paint-buckets. The star-system is bad for the stage because the minor parts are smothered and the situations distorted to give the favourite an orbit. It is bad for the motion pictures because it obscures the producer. While the leading actor is entitled to his glory, as are all the actors, their mannerisms should not overshadow the latest inspirations of the creator of the films.

The display of the name of the corporation is no substitute for giving the glory to the producer. An artistic photoplay is not the result of a military efficiency system. It is not a factory-made staple article, but the product of the creative force of one soul, the flowering of a spirit that has the habit of perpetually renewing itself.

37. The passage implies that photoplay:
- **A** is nothing more than mere hieroglyphic.
- **B** is all about moving objects rather than performing actors.
- **C** requires greater visual creativity than theatre.
- **D** objectifies actors.

38. The author's claim statement that "The key-words of the stage are passion and character; of the photoplay, splendour and speed" suggests that theatre:
- **A** represents internal responses while film, outward appearances.
- **B** represents human attributes while film, objects.
- **C** deals with drama while film, the setting.
- **D** deals with the slow authenticity of the human experience while film, visual spectacle.

39. In modern filmmaking, "hieroglyphic" in the passage would closely resemble:
- **A** a scenic design.
- **B** make up.
- **C** shots.
- **D** visual effects.

40. In modern-day language, "producer" in the passage would refer to:
- **A** a film director.
- **B** a production designer.
- **C** an executive producer.
- **D** a line producer.

41. Which of the following statements would best express the author's view towards the theatre and the silent film?
- **A** The theatre and the silent film are in direct contrast to each other.
- **B** These two forms compete to eradicate the other's art.
- **C** The silent film is a reaction to the theatre's limitations.
- **D** These two forms comprise what is half expressed in the other's medium.

42. Based on the passage, which could be inferred to describe the stage actor's performance as opposed to that of the movie actor's?
- **A** The stage actor embodies the emotions and the "fate" of the plot, while the movie actor is simply part of the images that fill in the plot.
- **B** The stage actor has to exaggerate his performance while the movie actor depends on the camera's visual play.
- **C** The stage actor is a better performer than the movie actor.
- **D** The stage actor shares his powerful performance with the rest of the cast while the movie actor is the star of the film.

Questions 43 – 47

Research Models of Conceptual Methodology and Critical Analysis

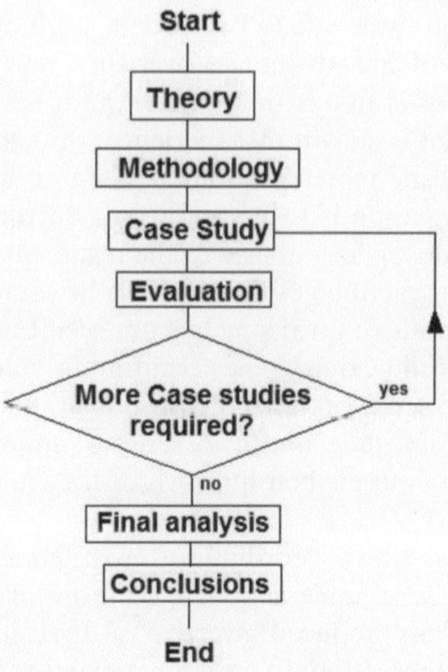

43. How does the "More Case Studies Required" yes-option function in the diagram?
- **A** As a necessary error in research protocol
- **B** As a balancing factor that avoids speculation
- **C** As an ad hoc modification of theory
- **D** As a feedback loop requiring more research

44. Using more Case Studies in theory is logically:
- **A** deductive.
- **B** inductive.
- **C** evidence-based.
- **D** a reservation or limitation.

45. Which of the following could be inferred to be included in the conclusions?
- **A** Theoretical Assumptions
- **B** Methodological Concerns
- **C** More Case Studies
- **D** Areas of Future Research

46. Which of the following could be inferred to be included in the methodology?
- **A** Scope of Study and Review of Literature
- **B** Areas of Future Research
- **C** Theoretical Assumptions
- **D** Limitations and Reservations

47. What would be the best critique of this model?
- **A** It proposes ad hoc examples to support theory.
- **B** Its "More Case Studies" is non-falsifying.
- **C** It avoids its own biases and prejudices.
- **D** It is too simplistic for complex phenomena.

Questions 48 – 54

The following is an excerpt from Aristotle's Poetics.

It is clear that the general origin of poetry was due to two causes, each of them part of human nature. Imitation is natural to man from childhood, one of his advantages over the lower animals being this, that he is the most imitative creature in the world, and learns at first by imitation. And it is also natural for all to delight in works of imitation. The truth of this second point is shown by experience: though the objects themselves may be painful to see, we delight to view the most realistic representations of them in art, the forms for example of the lowest animals and of dead bodies. The explanation is to be found in a further fact: to be learning something is the greatest of pleasures not only to the philosopher but also to the rest of mankind, however small their capacity for it; the reason of the delight in seeing the picture is that one is at the same time learning—gathering the meaning of things, e.g. that the man there is so-and-so; for if one has not seen the thing before, one's pleasure will not be in the picture as an imitation of it, but will be due to the execution or colouring or some similar cause. Imitation, then, being natural to us—as also the sense of harmony and rhythm, the metres being obviously species of rhythms—it was through their original aptitude, and by a series of improvements for the most part gradual on their first efforts, that they created poetry out of their improvisations.

Poetry, however, soon broke up into two kinds according to the differences of character in the individual poets; for the graver among them would represent noble actions, and those of noble personages; and the meaner sort the actions of the ignoble. The latter class produced invectives at first, just as others did hymns and panegyrics. In this poetry of invective its natural fitness brought an iambic metre into use; hence our present term 'iambic', because it was the metre of their 'iambs' or invectives against one another. The result was that the old poets became some of them writers of heroic and others of iambic verse. Homer's position, however, is peculiar: just as he was in the serious style the poet of poets, standing alone not only through the literary excellence, but also through the dramatic character of his imitations, so too he was the first to outline for us the general forms of Comedy by producing not a dramatic invective, but a dramatic picture of the Ridiculous; his Margites in fact stands in the same relation to our comedies as the Iliad and Odyssey to our tragedies. As soon, however, as Tragedy and Comedy appeared in the field, those naturally drawn to the one line of poetry became writers of comedies instead of iambs, and those naturally drawn to the other, writers of tragedies instead of epics, because these new modes of art were grander and of more esteem than the old.

It certainly began in improvisations—as did also Comedy; the one originating with the authors of the Dithyramb, the other with those of the phallic songs, which still survive as institutions in many of our cities. And its advance after that was little by little, through their improving on whatever they had before them at each stage. It was in fact only after a long series of changes that the movement of Tragedy stopped on its attaining to its natural form.

48. According to passage information, an iamb originally means:
- **A** a hymn.
- **B** an insult.
- **C** a foot.
- **D** a panegyric.

49. Based on passage information, poetry is:
- **A** a mimetic process.
- **B** an offshoot of Tragedy and Comedy.
- **C** a rhythmic improvisation.
- **D** tragedy in its natural form.

50. Which of these statements would most probably support Aristotle's idea of poetry?

A Poetry is an echo of the poet's soul.
B Poetry reflects reality.
C Poetry is saying something while meaning the other.
D Poetry is ordinary language raised to the Nth power.

51. Human beings find pleasure in works of imitation because:

A they are sources of knowledge.
B they delight in watching objects of pain and listening to words of insult.
C they contain moral lessons.
D it is in their nature to imitate.

52. Based on passage information, what is the author's attitude towards Comedy?

A Unbiased
B Amused
C Evaluative
D Critical

53. Which of the following scenarios would most probably serve as a good material for Tragedy?

A A bicycle champion amputating his leg stuck beneath an upturned truck
B A street orphan shot dead by the police after stealing bread for her homeless friends
C A military general donating his eyes to an enemy's son
D A black slave taking a bullet meant for the slave trader

54. If considered true, which of these statements is not consistent with Aristotle's ideas?

A Insects have mastered the art of imitation to protect themselves from predators.
B Poetry is an assault on ordinary language.
C Comedy is legitimate insult.
D Enjoying imitative works and learning are two distinct ends of the creative process.

UNIT 11

Questions 55 – 61

Consider the following passage and comments in answering the questions.

Some aspects of postmodern art concern self-consciousness of the art act itself, the laying bare of the devices used to construct the illusion or representation, and blurring the divisions between the audience and the art. For example, John Cage, a pianist and to some extent experimentalist in art, recorded only audience noise for one of his compositions: the shuffling about in seats, coughs, whispers, etc… all to some extent, what would be considered noise. His most famous work is the 4'33", *which he composed in 1952. This piece is performed in three movements without the musician hitting a single note for four minutes and thirty three seconds. The composition is supposed to consist of the sounds of the surroundings that the listener hears while it is performed.*

The following remarks are quoted from Cage himself:

Comment I

Wherever we are, what we hear is mostly noise. When we ignore it, it disturbs us. When we listen to it, we find it fascinating.

Comment II

People who are not artists often feel that artists are inspired. But if you work at your art you don't have time to be inspired.

Comment III

Ideas are one thing and what happens is another.

Comment IV

The grand thing about the human mind is that it can turn its own tables and see meaninglessness as ultimate meaning.

Comment V

Art's purpose is to sober and quiet the mind so that it is in accord with what happens.

Comment VI

The first question I ask myself when something doesn't seem to be beautiful is why do I think it's not beautiful. And very shortly you discover that there is no reason.

Comment VII

The highest purpose is to have no purpose at all. This puts one in accord with nature, in her manner of operation.

55. In Comment I, which of the following could be reasonably inferred about John Cage's view of music?
- **A** Music takes different forms.
- **B** Music is an affirmation of life.
- **C** Silence is music in itself.
- **D** The appreciation of music depends on how you listen to it.

56. Comments V and VII support the notion that the purpose of music is to:
A have no purpose at all.
B bring about internal order out of chaos.
C reveal the natural motion of life.
D liberate the listeners from artificial conventions.

57. How many of the comments would contradict the concept that art should be an expression of the artist's inner state rather than his or her subject?
A 4
B 2
C 3
D 1

58. Which of Comments I to VII is closely similar to the idea of "art for art's sake"?
A Comment II
B Comment IV
C Comment V
D Comment VII

Questions 59 – 61 relate to the pictures or the comments, whichever is applicable.

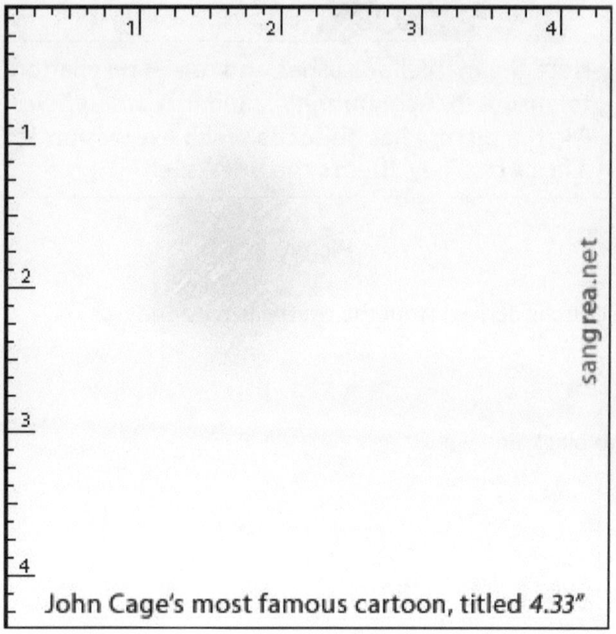

Picture 1

59. Which among Comments I to VII does Picture 1 relate with?
A Comment III
B Comment IV
C Comment VI
D Comment VII

60. In relation to the comments, what makes Picture 1 humorous?
A Its self-referentiality
B There is nothing there, except the two axes.
C It mocks the pretensions of such notions.
D All of the above

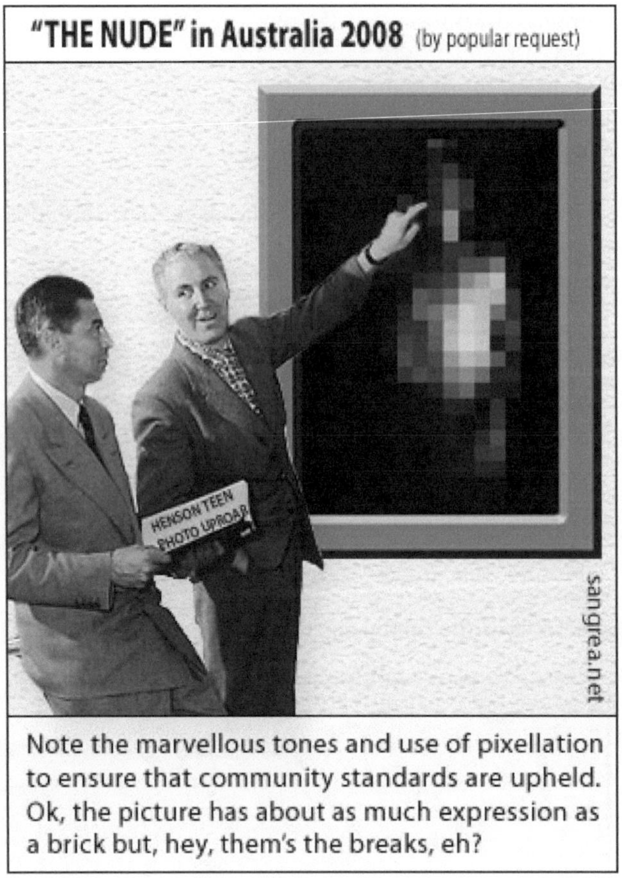

Picture 2

61. The humour in this picture is derived from the overbearing standards of:

A censorship.
B representation.
C traditional art.
D colour contrast to black and white.

Question 62

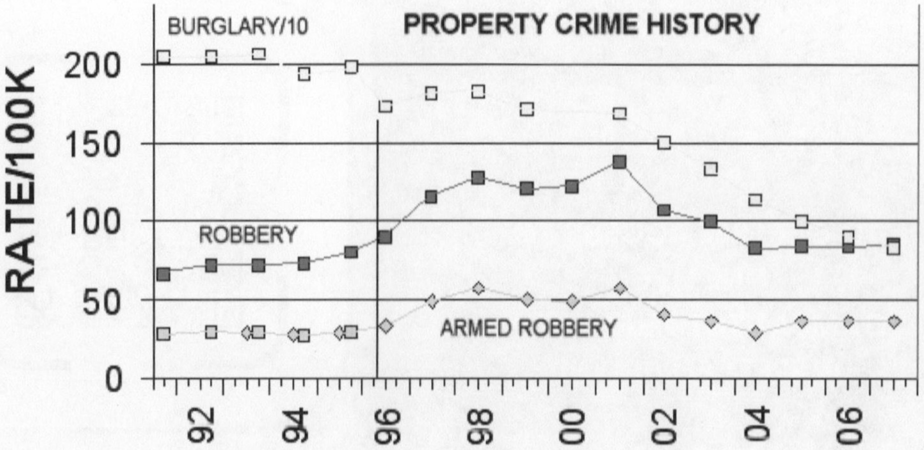

Figure 1. Property Crime History in Australia

62. Which of the following would make the best generalisation concerning Australian crime rates based on Figure 1?

A The decline of burglary, over the years, corresponds to a rise in robbery.
B The rates for robbery and armed robbery rose faster after 1996, and stayed higher for a few years.
C All three types of crime do not decline after 1993.
D It appears that a short term increase in armed robbery occurred after 2002.